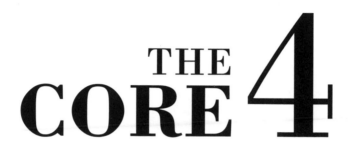

THE CORE 4

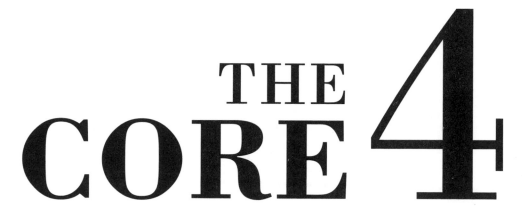

THE CORE 4

EMBRACE YOUR BODY, OWN YOUR POWER

Steph Gaudreau

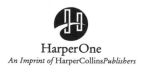

HarperOne

An Imprint of HarperCollinsPublishers

HarperOne

FIRST EDITION

Designed by Kris Tobiassen
Fitness photographs by Richwell Correa
Food photographs by Stephanie Gaudreau

Library of Congress Cataloging-in-Publication Data has been applied for.

ISBN 978-0-06-285975-4

19 20 21 22 23 LSC 10 9 8 7 6 5 4 3 2 1

WAITER WALKS—*3 sets of 50 feet with each arm*

Stand with your feet under your hips and hold light- to moderate-weight dumbbells in each hand. Press your right dumbbell up toward the ceiling, actively pushing through your shoulder and keeping your right arm close to your head. Then walk with the dumbbell overhead. Pull your ribs down instead of flaring them out. Repeat the movements with your left arm.

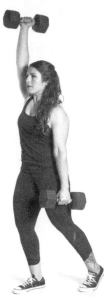

SEATED SIDE TWISTS—*3 sets of 8 reps on each side*

Sit on the floor with your knees bent, your feet flat on the floor, and a dumbbell held in both hands at chest height. Lean back, bringing your feet off the floor, and slowly twist your body to the right as you move the dumbbell toward your right hip. Keep your sit bones on the floor. Then rotate your body slowly to the left, moving the dumbbell toward your left hip. Keep the weight close to your body as you rotate from side to side.

The ultimate goal is full range of motion. Missing internal rotation as part of your range of motion isn't good either!

Day 10 Challenge: Work Out

Again, movements from Week 1 make a dynamic warm-up. Complete all sets and reps of each movement before moving on to the next.

Make sure to track your sleep today.

LEVEL 1

SUITCASE DEADLIFTS—*4 sets of 10 reps*

Position your feet hip width apart and hold dumbbells or kettlebells next to your feet. Engage your core, squeeze your glutes, and come to a standing position by trying to push the floor away with your legs instead of lifting with your back. Keep your spine aligned throughout the movement, and keep the weights close to your body. Then hinge forward at the hip and return to the starting position. Be sure to keep your toes from lifting off the floor throughout the movement.

Pro Tip

» *To make it harder,* use a barbell.

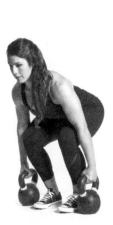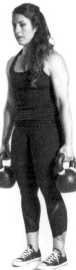

ALTERNATING DUMBBELL SHOULDER PRESSES—*3 sets of 8 reps with each arm*

Stand with your feet under your hips and with dumbbells in both hands held at shoulder height, with your knuckles facing your shoulders. Engage your core, squeeze your butt, and keep your neck neutral as you actively push up through the shoulder to raise one dumbbell toward the ceiling. Keep your arm close to your head. Also, pull your ribs down instead of flaring them out. Lower the dumbbell and repeat the movements with the opposite arm.

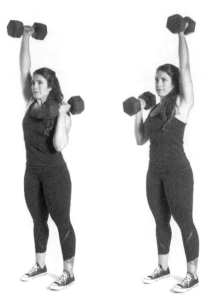

Pro Tip

» *To make it harder,* press both dumbbells up at the same time or use a barbell.

PLANKS—*4 sets of 20 seconds*

Lie on the floor facedown with your hands next to your chest and your elbows close to your sides. Take a breath and push your body up onto your toes and hands, engaging your core and keeping your body in a straight line. Don't stick your butt up in the air or let your hips sag. Hold this position, breathing normally.

Pro Tip

» *To make it harder,* add weight to your back, or lift one leg off the floor.

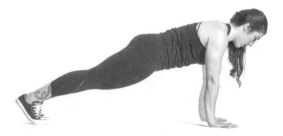

MOUNTAIN CLIMBERS—*5 reps per leg*

Get on the floor in the plank position, with your hands shoulder width apart. Engage your core as you quickly pull one knee toward your chest, just touching your foot to the floor before extending that leg back again. Repeat the movement with the opposite leg. Continue to alternate legs.

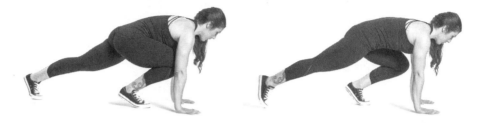

SQUATS—*12 reps*

Stand with your feet under your hips. Keeping your feet flat on the floor, engage your core as you push your hips back and bend your knees, lowering until your thighs are a little lower than parallel to the floor (or as low as feels comfortable). Go as low as you can while keeping a neutral spine. Your knees should track over your feet, and your chest should remain up. Then return to the starting position.

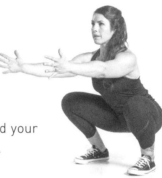

DAY 14: EMPTY BATTERY

You're two weeks into the Core 4 program. How does your body feel? With six workouts under your belt, you may already notice a difference, especially when it comes to feeling more like a badass. And the more workouts you do, the more you'll own that. But for today's challenge, I want you to slow down a bit.

When you think of your energy, your thoughts might automatically drift to topics like sleep or recovery practices. You might even think that recharging your energy takes many hours or involves difficult tasks.

LEVEL 2

BARBELL BACK SQUATS—*5 sets of 5 reps at RPE 6*

Stand with a barbell resting across the meaty back of your shoulders, called the trapezius muscles, and held in an overhand grip. Don't let the barbell rest on your neck bones. Inhale, engage your core, squeeze your glutes, and hinge at the hip before bending your knees to lower your butt toward the floor until your thighs are parallel to the floor or slightly lower. Keep your neck neutral and your chest high, then return to the starting position, exhaling on the way up.

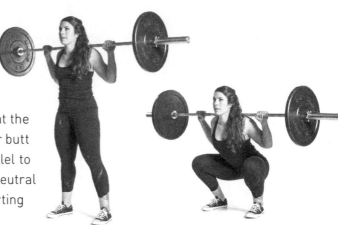

BARBELL POWER CLEANS—*3 sets of 3 reps at RPE 6*

Stand with your feet slightly wider than hip width apart and with a barbell on the floor in front of your feet. Hinge at the hips and grab the barbell overhand with your hands positioned just outside your hips. Lift it to your thighs, then push with your legs and jump as you bend your elbows to flip the bar up and shrug it to your shoulders. The power comes from your legs driving the bar up rather than pulling it with your arms. Stand in a partial squat with your knees slightly bent. Pause briefly, then return the bar to the floor.

Pro Tip

» *To make it harder,* use an unbalanced object like a sandbag, or receive the weight in a full squat clean.

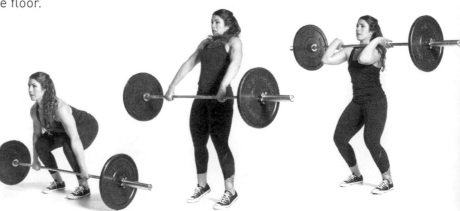

ALTERNATING DUMBBELL SHOULDER PRESSES—*3 sets of 8 reps with each arm*

Stand with your feet under your hips and with dumbbells in both hands held at shoulder height, with your knuckles facing your shoulders. Engage your core, squeeze your butt, and keep your neck neutral as you actively push up through the shoulder to raise one dumbbell toward the ceiling. Keep your arm close to your head. Also, pull your ribs down instead of flaring them out. Lower the dumbbell and repeat the movements with the opposite arm.

Pro Tip

» *To make it harder,* press both dumbbells up at the same time or use a barbell.

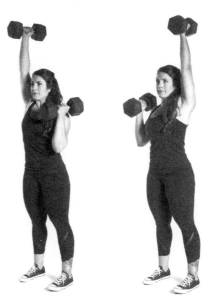

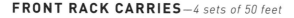

FRONT RACK CARRIES—*4 sets of 50 feet*

Stand with your feet under your hips and hold a pair of dumbbells directly in front of your chest. Engage your core and walk forward, taking normal-size steps and keeping the weights steady and close to your chest with your elbows pinned to your sides.

Pro Tip

» *To make it harder,* substitute a barbell for the dumbbells.

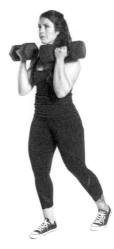

BARBELL SHOULDER PRESSES —*3 sets of 5 reps at RPE 6*

Stand with your feet under your hips and holding a barbell across the front of your shoulders with an overhand grip. Your hands should be slightly wider than shoulder width apart. Engage your core, press the barbell toward the ceiling. Maintain a neutral posture and pull your ribs down instead of flaring them out. Return to the starting position.

PULL-UPS —*4 sets of 5 reps*

Stand under a pull-up bar with your hands gripping the bar underhand or overhand (your choice) and shoulder width apart. Your thumbs should be wrapped all the way around the bar. Inhale as you engage your core and pull your body up until your chin clears the bar. Keep your neck neutral—don't crane your chin over the bar. Then lower back to the starting position with control to protect your shoulders.

Pro Tips

» *To make it easier*, secure a band around the bar and place your feet in it to reduce the amount of weight you're pulling up. Or start at the top of the pull-up position and then lower yourself down instead of doing the complete rep.

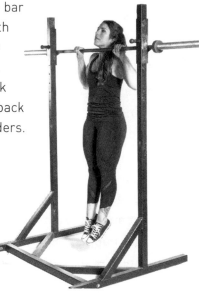

PULL-UPS—*4 sets of 6 reps*

Stand under a pull-up bar with your hands gripping the bar underhand or overhand (your choice) and shoulder width apart. Your thumbs should be wrapped all the way around the bar. Inhale as you engage your core and pull your body up until your chin clears the bar. Keep your neck neutral—don't crane your chin over the bar. Then lower back to the starting position with control to protect your shoulders.

Pro Tips

» *To make it easier,* secure a band around the bar and place your feet in it to reduce the amount of weight you're pulling up. Or start at the top of the pull-up position and then lower yourself down instead of doing the complete rep.

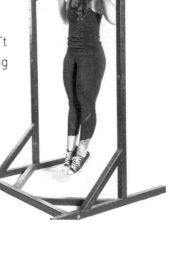

L SITS—*3 sets*

Sit on the floor with your legs extended in front of you and your hands gripping dumbbells on the floor next to your hips. Inhale and engage your core as you lift your butt off the floor, supporting your bodyweight on your hands. Hold for 15 to 30 seconds, then lower to the floor.

Pro Tip

» *To make it easier,* lift one leg off the floor—it can be either bent or straight.

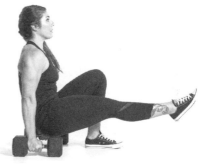

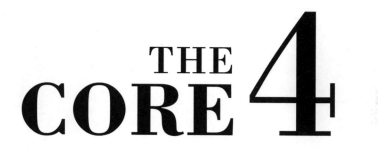

THE CORE 4

EMBRACE YOUR BODY, OWN YOUR POWER

Steph Gaudreau

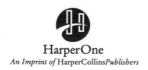

HarperOne
An Imprint of HarperCollins*Publishers*

HarperOne

THE CORE 4. Copyright © 2019 by Stephanie Gaudreau. All rights reserved. Printed in the United States of America. No part of this book may be used or reproduced in any manner whatsoever without written permission except in the case of brief quotations embodied in critical articles and reviews. For information, address HarperCollins Publishers, 195 Broadway, New York, NY 10007.

HarperCollins books may be purchased for educational, business, or sales promotional use. For information, please email the Special Markets Department at SPsales@harpercollins.com.

FIRST EDITION

Designed by Kris Tobiassen
Fitness photographs by Richwell Correa
Food photographs by Stephanie Gaudreau

Library of Congress Cataloging-in-Publication Data has been applied for.

ISBN 978-0-06-285975-4

19 20 21 22 23 LSC 10 9 8 7 6 5 4 3 2 1

For Laurie and Ruth,
the two strongest women I know

*Sweet Potato Breakfast Bowls
(page 262)*

Savory Ham and Egg Cups
(page 259)

Steak Cobb Salad with Southwestern Ranch Dressing (page 267)

Chopped Broccoli Salad (page 269)

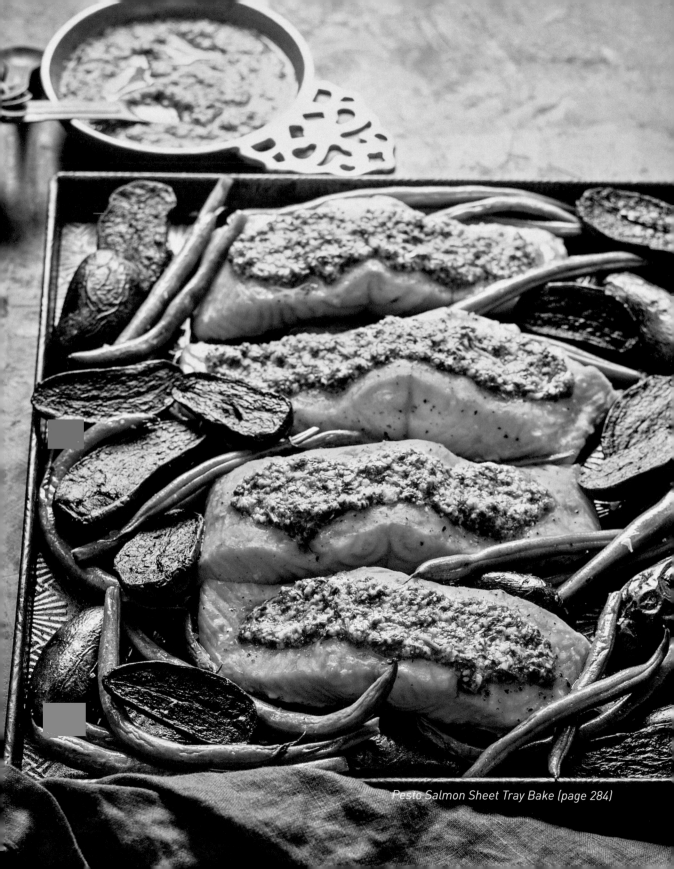

Pesto Salmon Sheet Tray Bake (page 284)

Hearty Tuscan Kale Soup
(page 264)

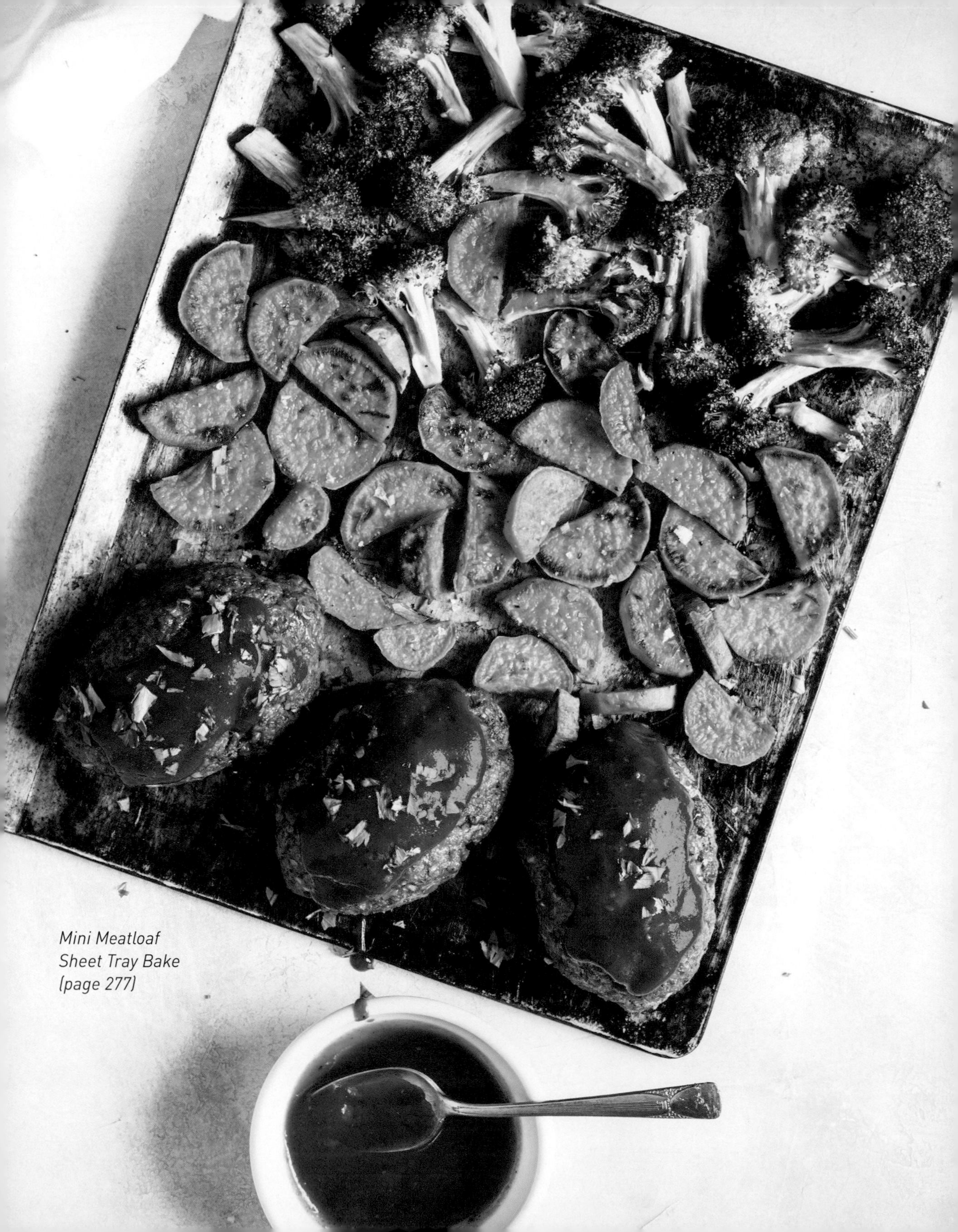

Mini Meatloaf
Sheet Tray Bake
(page 277)

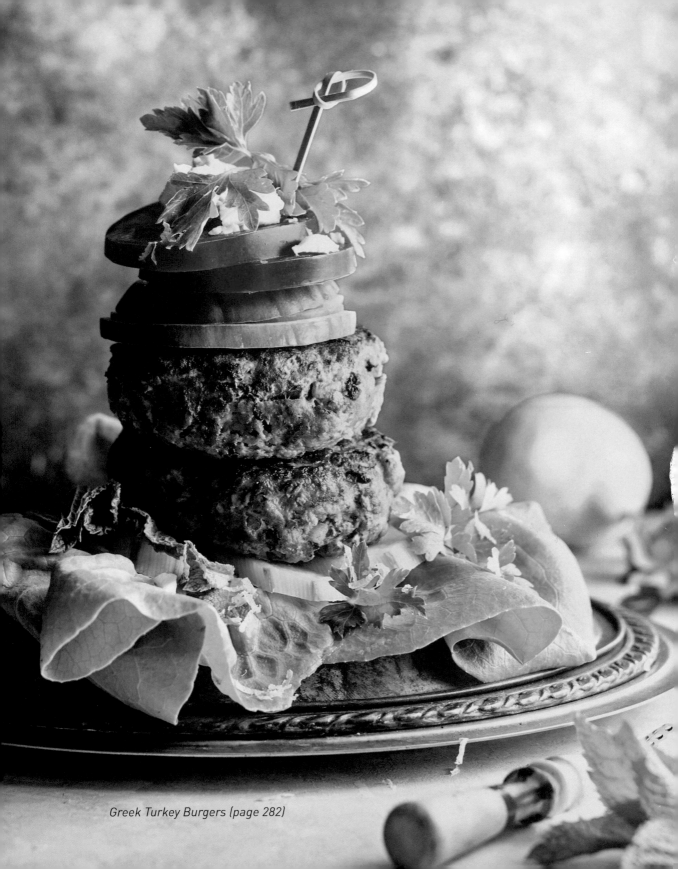

Greek Turkey Burgers (page 282)

CONTENTS

Take Your Power Back

I have a vision . . . a vision that someday little girls will grow up into strong women who love their bodies, know their worth, and take up space without the pressure of diets, the scale, or exercise as punishment.

Building that world starts with you and me—today. By refusing to let your weight measure your worth. By nourishing your body. By letting your intuition guide you. By taking your power back. If you follow the simple (but challenging!) program I offer you in this book, and commit to fiercely and ruthlessly embracing yourself for the next 30 days, I guarantee you'll start feeling energetic, active, confident, strong, resilient, and ready to change the world.

Okay, let's back up for a second. I understand you may not be in change-the-world mode yet. In fact, you may not even be in get-out-of-bed mode yet. However, I'm going to guess you picked up this book because you're ready to try something different. You may even be ready to question conventional wisdom and make a big, 180-degree turn. Wherever you are, you're ready to act and to start on this path to your best health—and your fullest life.

If you're unhappy with your body—and most women are—you probably still believe that if you can just make your body perfect, life will be all rainbows and unicorns. You'll be free of the negative thoughts you've battled for years. Your feelings of unworthiness will disappear.

While the never-ending quest to shrink your body and make yourself small is tempting, it leads only to disappointment. It requires focusing on the physical without healing your inner self—the person who sometimes feels worthless, forgotten, and like she's never "enough." And the diet industry is there to kick you when you're down, needling your biggest insecurities, exposing your vulnerabilities, and then swooping in with a "solution." Take this pill. Do this 1,200-calorie diet plan. Suffer through exercises you hate.

Well, fuck all that. Women are tired and fed up, and they want off that roller-coaster ride for good.

The path to health is multifaceted, but at its core is the need to nourish yourself both inside and out. This is how to achieve true wellness in mind, body, and spirit. It doesn't mean that life is then perfect. Rather, it means you have the gumption to really live, to do and experience and create. To be big and bold in your own way. And to weather life's challenges with grace and resilience.

You've got to take a stand and do things differently if you want to thrive in this world. And I'm happy to tell you that thriving means expanding—mentally, physically, emotionally. It means getting outside your comfort zone. It means taking action even when you're scared. It means questioning the status quo and doing the work to unlearn the habits that no longer serve you. It means having the confidence to wear whatever you want in public—shorts, a tank top, or a bathing suit—and realize you don't have to make anyone else comfortable about your body. It means waking up every day refreshed and ready to tackle whatever comes your way. It means taking care of yourself from a place of respect and compassion. It means having a strong, capable, body; glowing skin, hair, and nails; a positive, uplifted mood; stable energy levels; awesome digestion; few food cravings; and a healthy sex drive (*meow*).

Before I tell you more about the Core 4 program, I want to tell you about me. When it comes to nutrition, fitness, weight loss, and athletic performance, I have seen it all, heard it all, and tried it all. As a Nutritional Therapy Consultant and fitness coach, I have identified, tested, and fine-tuned the elements of the Core 4. I've touched millions with my work online—through recipes, podcasts, and fitness tips—and worked directly with thousands of health seekers.

But before I did all that, I was like a lot of women. Pretty much all my life I hated my body, especially my thighs. I hated the fact that I felt so much bigger than other girls. I thought the answer to finding happiness and self-acceptance must be to get smaller. So I became obsessed with controlling my food. I subsisted on Diet Coke, cucumber sandwiches, celery sticks, fat-free cheese, and those green 100-calorie snack packs. I spent more than a decade on an intense quest to lose weight. It's all I thought about. I tried every terrible diet—everything from the cabbage soup diet to just eating as little as possible. My goal with food and exercise was to shrink myself. Every morning I'd pinch my inner thighs to see how fat I was.

I was miserable. I struggled to wake up in the morning, chugged caffeine to get me through the day, and couldn't fall asleep at night. I was hypoglycemic, bloated all the time, and constantly in a bad mood, and I would snap at people for no reason. I guess you could call me a hangry bitch because that's how I felt: out of control but clueless about how to stop it. By the time I was in my early thirties, I thought fatigue, digestive problems, irrational moods, and bad skin were just what my life was going to be all about.

In early 2010, friends introduced me to a paleo way of eating. I figured I had nothing left to lose. I started focusing on real, whole foods, like animal protein, veggies, fruit, and healthy fats. And though I ate according to a strict list of foods (for the record, I wasn't eating nearly enough carbs because I thought that would help me "lean out"), for the first time in years I didn't count calories or obsess about my portions. Within a few months I started to notice some changes. My skin began to clear up. I slept more soundly and woke up refreshed, and I had more energy, but I was still miserable about how my body looked and about my weight, even though I was living in a thin body.

Desperate for change, I started training for off-road triathlons after several years of competitive mountain biking. I ramped up my workouts, I wasn't eating enough, and everything seemed to spiral out of control like a car-crash video playing in slow motion. I stepped on a scale at the end of race season and saw that my weight was at a lifetime low. Yet I still thought I was too heavy. To make things worse, my second marriage was falling apart. The long hours of training gave me the perfect excuse to bike, swim, and run myself to numbness. After a weekend spent racing at Lake Tahoe, I posed for a photo at Eagle Falls. I distinctly remember looking at the photo right after it was taken and thinking I'd never looked bigger, sending me into a silent scream. This was my rock bottom.

What I didn't realize then—and what I would slowly come to understand over the next few years—is that health and happiness aren't found on the bathroom scale. Seeing what was missing and where I was stuck is easy looking back. But at the time, when I was sitting in the soup, boiling away, I couldn't get my head above the surface long enough to figure out what those missing pieces were.

Just two short months later, after a friend dared me to do a CrossFit workout in my garage, I joined a gym and learned to lift weights. **With my hands on a barbell, I felt at home.** I was free to take up more space in a way that felt right for me, not according to society's expectations. I took my power back, and it was intoxicating. For the first time ever, I started focusing on what my body could *do* instead of what it looked like. Lifting weights changed my mindset. Instead of drifting off in my head and obsessing over my body the way I typically would, I learned to direct my energy and stay present. My confidence blossomed, and I finally felt comfortable in my own skin. I thought about what I wanted to do with my life. I felt . . . free. There's something exhilarating about approaching a heavy weight, lifting it, and thinking, *Hmm, I wonder what else I can do!* To me, squatting became the ultimate metaphor for life: When the weight of the world is on my shoulders, I know I can still rise up. I can overcome.

In the year that followed, I started personalizing my food to my needs and left the strict list behind. It took some tuning in to my body and trial and error, no doubt, but once I got it dialed in, my health issues all but vanished. That, in combination with building my physical strength and shedding the chains of my body obsession, opened up my energy to other things, like writing about my experiences of food and exercise with the entire world on a blog. Though I was still teaching high school full time, I developed a passion for sharing how I had overcome my challenges by eating nourishing food and strength training. As I figured out this powerful combination and healed my relationship with food and my body, I knew I had a duty, a mission, to share it with others.

In 2013, three years after embarking on what I now call my Core 4 journey, I left the classroom to devote myself fully to coaching women through the same process that had changed my life. I continued to research and experiment with how to build a resilient body, refining and expanding my framework to include more than food—what I call the gateway drug to wellness—and movement. But you know what? Even if those are great on-ramps to get started, they aren't the complete picture. True resil-

ience also takes rest, recovery, stress management, and, above all else, mindset. It requires mental, emotional, and spiritual strength in addition to physical strength. And frankly, resilience transcends the scope of this book; it also encompasses issues like social identities and access to resources.

I recently made the intentional shift away from producing just a "food blog," because I realized that providing recipes alone was doing my community a disservice. In a complex world where women are under so much pressure, my aim is to support them in all aspects of their health—the hard, fierce, relentless parts and the soft, soulful, surrendering parts. In other words, my support may start with food, but it sure as hell doesn't end there. If my vision of a powerful resilience is going to become a reality, it'll take moving from, as the saying goes, me to we, from shrinking our bodies to expanding ourselves and taking up all the space we need. That is why I developed the Core 4 program. Consider this book your road map for that journey.

THE CORE 4 PROGRAM

Why can you, your friends, and every woman in the world benefit from the Core 4 program? Let me set the stage: There's a prevailing belief that to change your health and your body, you have to hate on yourself. That the way to make progress is to be hard on yourself, to berate yourself when you mess up. For only a very small number of the women I've worked with, this "negative motivation" gets them somewhere. But for the vast majority, it eventually fails, sometimes spectacularly. When I ask women why they take this approach, the answer is almost always a resounding "If I'm not hard on myself, I'm afraid I'll stop caring." Let's nip that in the bud right now. Releasing self-hatred and punishment, dieting and restriction, doesn't mean you've given up or stopped caring. Having discipline to nourish your body and make choices from a place of self-compassion and self-respect is different from trying to hate your body into submission. You picked up this book because what you've done before hasn't worked. Take this journey with me and learn a new way.

You may be ready to show up with courage and to commit to living a bigger life. And if you're not ready quite yet, I can guarantee you will be by the end of this book. The Core 4 is about cultivating resilience—the ability to bounce back stronger after shitty things happen (because they will, eventually)—instead of living small, isolating

yourself from challenges and new experiences. This program is equal parts ethos and rallying cry.

Being strong is about taking action even when you're scared, because growth happens on that razor-thin edge between your comfort zone and the unknown. It involves intentionally examining your relationship with food, movement, rest, and self-care. Strength is as much about overcoming obstacles and pushing through your sticking points as giving yourself grace and space to breathe and be. Being fierce means standing up and saying, "Yes, my self-worth extends light-years beyond my physical body." Being strong is defining your life on your terms and owning your inner power.

In essence, a strong, fierce, resilient woman is someone ready to show up bigger in every way because she's fucking tired of making herself small.

Welcome, we've been waiting for you. You are home.

Commit to the Core 4 for 30 days, and each day you'll learn about and take actions that will help you grow stronger in body, mind, and spirit.

The key is to build a robust foundation, a comprehensive approach that targets four elements of wellness—what I call the Core 4 pillars. These pillars work for anyone, regardless of age, experience, or fitness level, and already they have been proven effective by people who have followed the Core 4 program online. The description of each pillar may sound simple, but each one is necessary for the healthiest version of you.

Pillar 1: Eat Nourishing Foods
Pillar 2: Move with Intention
Pillar 3: Recharge Your Energy
Pillar 4: Empower Your Mind

You won't build health by focusing on only one pillar. Most women struggle to make lasting changes because their foundation is shaky, based on perfecting one of these pillars while neglecting the others. Soon everything crumbles, and they're back at square one, feeling frustrated and hopeless. For long-term success, you must build and balance the Core 4 pillars *together*, a little at a time, by making small, manageable changes. This stabilizes the foundation that supports your strength, health, and confidence. Consistency, not perfection, is the name of the game.

At the time of writing this book, more than one thousand people have experienced—and had their lives changed by—the Core 4 program. They know firsthand how powerful this framework is.

Michelle, age forty, says: The [Core 4 program] was one of the best gifts I have ever given to myself. I was unsure about it at first, but it changed everything for me. It didn't just address healthy eating and exercise but dove deeper into renewing your energy and changing the way you think about yourself. It made me feel more positive about the body I have and how far I have come on my journey.

Abby, age thirty-seven, had tried just about every diet before she found the Core 4: I had been hopping from meal plan to meal plan, workout plan to workout plan, quick fix to quick fix for so long. I call this challenge the "challenge to end all challenges," because Steph has empowered me with the tools and knowledge I need to live a holistically healthy life. I felt for a long time that I was doing everything perfectly—eating low-calorie and working out six days a week for an hour, sometimes two. I was unknowingly beating myself into the ground and sacrificing energy I could have been using to enjoy life. Through Steph's gentle, and sometimes tough, love, I learned how backward this all-or-nothing thinking is!

WHAT TO EXPECT

Now let's get to the good stuff.

What can you expect from the Core 4 program? In part I, you'll learn the fundamentals of the Core 4 pillars and the rationale behind them. Then in part II you'll find a 30-day, day-by-day program to help you practice new habits with me as your guide. Even though this is a proven 30-day framework, this isn't a one-size-fits-all plan. I want you to personalize it. So before you begin the program, you'll fill out a Personal Pillar Plan, which will take into account your goals, strengths, and areas for improvement, as well as a Health Tracker, which will give you an objective measure of your overall health. Later in the book you'll also find recipes for all the meals you'll be enjoying during these next 30 days, plus guides to the movements in your daily workouts and all the motivation, advice, and guidance you'll need to keep going. You'll have some freedom with this pro-

gram, because independence and choice matter, but you'll find boundaries as well—I don't want you jumping down every rabbit hole or wandering in the wilderness of the "health space" forever.

Shifting your focus from weight *loss* to health *gain* and building health from the inside out may sound counterintuitive. But emphasizing what you're adding to your life instead of fretting about everything you're giving up is a powerful paradigm shift. Instead of shrinking—both literally and figuratively—**you'll work toward expanding your potential, your health, and your confidence even while you experience the changes in your body that you want.**

By the end of this kick-start month, I have every confidence that you'll have a stronger, more badass body; a new sense of confidence in yourself and your ability to pursue your dreams; closer, more meaningful relationships with your family and friends; and better overall health. Plus, you'll possess all the tools you need to keep going on your journey, changing them up as needed.

I wrote this book to reach people. Maybe you're coming into this with a specific goal, like losing twenty pounds. I get that. But I'll show you how to do it in a way that propels you forward and feels, dare I say, easy and fun, instead of hard and punishing. Whoever decided that getting healthier has to suck is just crazy. Food and energy and mindset and movement are all interrelated. Instead of thinking in a straight line, imagine a web where everything is connected. Every element touches, supports, and feeds back into your overall health and happiness.

I know what it's like to not feel like yourself—yet feel totally helpless when it comes to addressing it. This book lays out a path for you to move forward without losing your way. It's the book I wish I'd had when I embarked on my health journey ten years ago. I understand how challenging this journey can be (hello—I've been in your shoes!), but I won't let you slip back into the comfort zone of doing what you've always done.

My job as your nutrition expert, coach, and motivator over the course of your Core 4 journey is to call out bullshit when I see it—and to reflect your infinite goodness, worth, and potential back to you. I'm here to believe in you even when you don't fully believe in yourself. I'm here to spur you to try new things and to forget the conventional wisdom that doesn't work. For change to happen, you're going to have to take action.

That action starts now. For your body, your happiness, and your biggest, boldest, fiercest life.

PART I

THE CORE 4 FRAMEWORK

Eat Nourishing Foods

Let me ask you something: How do you feel? Do you feel strong, confident, well rested, and ready to tackle any challenge? Or do you feel fatigued, out of shape, overwhelmed, irritable, and dissatisfied with your body . . . even your life?

If you're like most women I work with, you feel the latter. You're unhappy with yourself and hope that losing weight, reaching a specific number on the scale, and getting smaller will make you happier, sexier, more successful, more satisfied—fill in the blank. But if reaching your goals has meant getting on a diet, the only other option you have is to be *off* the diet, and so begins the cycle of misery, frustration, and, eventually, another diet.

Whenever I hear or see diet commercials or ads online, I can't help but pick up on the snarky, condescending subtexts and the undertone of guilt and shame. Movies and television love to reduce women to simplistic stereotypes obsessed with pushing salad around on our plates. The messages to shrink are everywhere. It's no wonder the average woman who diets internalizes these messages until literally her own voice says the same things.

Deep down, we know dieting doesn't work, but when there isn't an alternative and losing weight feels like a lifelong ritual, it's easy to feel alone, overwhelmed, and disempowered. Everything we've been sold is that changing our health has to suck. Why do we keep swallowing this bullshit? (Rhetorical question.)

Embarking on your Core 4 journey means thinking about what you've internalized, peeling back the layers, and realizing that you get to rewrite the story. In short, **it's time to redefine your relationship with food**.

Diets promise that if you change your weight—your outside appearance—you will finally be happy inside. But it's not that simple. In fact, that's completely backward. I'm here to show you how to build lasting, sustainable inside-out health while treating yourself with kindness. The women I've worked with feel more energetic, vibrant, powerful, content, comfortable, confident in—even proud of—their bodies, and themselves, than they have in years . . . sometimes *ever*. And they do this without counting calories, restricting food, or using exercise as punishment.

How is this possible? By focusing on *gaining health*. Everything you're likely to read about dieting concentrates on losing weight, cutting back, depriving yourself, and shrinking your body. (Those don't even feel good when you read them, do they?) It's time to move on to a new way of thinking. You'll gain health by eating foods that nourish and satisfy you because you respect your body. You'll also build strength, recharge your batteries, and examine how you see the world . . . all components of the Core 4 pillars. And as you do this, you'll build your health from the inside out, live bigger, and expand your possibilities. How good will it feel to free yourself from a lifetime of micromanaging your body?

Allow me to point out a truth about bodyweight that nobody wants to admit: weight loss doesn't automatically equal better health. Some women need to gain muscle to be healthier. Some need to improve their blood sugar. Some need to fix their digestion. Some need to reduce their stress level. If you separate yourself from the number on the scale, I bet you can think of some things besides your weight that you'd like to improve. Better sleep? Clearer skin? More energy? Positive attitude? Greater sex drive? As you gain health, over time your body comes to an optimal, healthy weight *for you*. In other words, **weight loss is often an outcome of better health, not the cause**. Another unpopular truth? Even if you dramatically improve your health for the better in every way, the scale still may not show you what you expect to see. In the immortal words of *Frozen*'s Elsa, "Let it go!" And I'll add my corollary: If weighing yourself causes you more stress than peace of mind, stop using the scale. It's not a required tool for improving your health. If it isn't working for you, you have permission to get rid of it! You don't have any more time or energy to waste playing mental gymnastics with the

scale. It measures how much gravity is pulling down on your body. It doesn't always show you an accurate picture about health, and it certainly doesn't tell you your worth. The world is waiting for your powerful self to show up with all your gifts.

Typical diets come with a long list of foods to never eat again—usually all the really fun ones, right?! The Core 4 program isn't a diet, and while it comes with what I call a "Nourishing Foods Framework" to achieve the best results, which you'll find later in this chapter (pages 34–35), there will be no calorie counting, macronutrient logging, freaking out about fats and carbs, or starting the whole program over again if you ate something "off limits." This isn't a test of will. It's not a measure of how "good" you are because you followed some rules. There are no rewards for adhering to the most restrictive diet possible.

Let's pause, take a deep breath, and feel the burden of every insane diet rule you've ever followed melt away.

This first pillar in the Core 4 program is all about eating nourishing foods. That means eating

> nutrient-dense, real, whole foods;
>
> a balance of macronutrients in amounts that leave you feeling satisfied and energized;
>
> foods rich in vitamins, minerals, and fiber that look like they came from nature, not a factory;
>
> and the best quality foods within your means.

It also means honoring your unique needs, goals, and taste buds. It doesn't mean eating perfectly, but it does mean eating like you give a damn.

Eating nourishing foods means taking an additive, not a restrictive, approach. Elimination diets—in which you remove problematic foods for a few weeks, then reintroduce them to test how they affect you—have their merits. In fact, doing an elimination was how I discovered that cow dairy and I aren't friends. However, when I talk about a "restrictive" approach, I mean the common diets that tell you to take away all "bad" things—fat, salt, sugar, meat—and never eat them again. As if getting healthier means eating as little as possible with as little enjoyment as possible. In this restriction mode, you muscle through for a week or two and then give up when willpower disappears. With

Dieting by the Numbers

Dieting is big business in the United States—to the tune of more than $60 *billion* every year. And yet consider these statistics:

» More than 100 million people launch at least one diet every year.

» The average dieter starts a new diet four to five times a year.

» On any given day, 45 percent of women and 25 percent of men are dieting.

» Eighty-five percent of dieters and those who buy weight-loss products and services are women.

» Ninety-five percent of diets fail.

» Most dieters will regain any lost weight within the next one to five years.

» Seventy-five percent of women have unhealthy thoughts, feelings, or behaviors related to food and/or their bodies.

Sources: ABC News, Council on Size and Weight Discrimination, and ScienceDaily.

the Core 4, you'll take an additive approach instead, focusing on adding nutrient-dense, satiating, and—dare I say—delicious foods. The idea is that by adding nutrient-dense foods, you'll begin to crowd out some of the less nutritious ones over time. Healthier eating is sustainable when you have the most flexibility and options, not the least. For example, maybe you decide to add a veggie to your breakfast plate each day. That's very different from avoiding all carbs.

Even the words you use may change: "I *get to eat* avocado with my eggs" instead of "I *can't have* sugar." Which *feels* better to you? This additive approach lets you play, experiment, and learn how to eat better—while eating foods you actually enjoy. Sure, there are some processed foods you'll be better off without, but you'll be so busy focusing on all the delectable foods you get to eat that you won't miss them all that much. And on the random occasion when you do eat that donut, you're going to choose it, savor it, own the outcomes (if any), and move the hell on with your life instead of drowning in food guilt. This approach empowers you with regard to your food choices and allows you to flex your intuition muscle and start listening to your body.

It's worth noting that there's no one definitive list of foods that will work for everyone. A bioindividual approach to nutrition means valuing your unique needs, likes and dislikes, and even culture when it comes to food. Maybe you hate the taste of kale, you're allergic to eggs, or rice is a staple food in your culture. Honor those things. Take them into consideration as you move through the program, and look for an opportunity to add color, variety, and quality to your food when possible.

With that in mind, consider the framework in this chapter as a guide, not an exact prescription. Your best mix will be different from anyone else's. Because it's impossible to give an exact list of foods that works for all people, I'll be sticking to general recommendations instead of taking nerdy deep dives into specific topics like lectins, FODMAPs, and autoimmune protocols. Above all, if you continue to struggle with specific nutrition issues, consider working one-on-one with a qualified professional.

A talk about nourishing foods wouldn't be complete without considering how you best deal with change. You might be someone who thrives on gradual change that happens slowly over time. On the flip side, you might be a rip-off-the-Band-Aid kind of person who would rather get change over with and start with a clean slate. Neither method is wrong. If you're more comfortable with small chunks of change, commit to that. Swap out sweet potato noodles for pasta. Add egg yolks back into your omelets. Those small changes add up!

What makes a food nourishing? Every food can be broken down into several components, such as its calorie content; its macronutrient content (whether it has protein, carbs, fats, or a combination of these); its micronutrient content (the vitamins and minerals it contains); and other elements like water and fiber content. When I consider the nourishing value of a food, I look at the big picture of all of these parts. Most diets consider calorie counting or removing an entire food group as the be-all and end-all. There's a tendency to want to align with one camp and be dogmatic about how to eat. I want you to leave rigidity behind and instead consider *all* the criteria I just mentioned when moving forward.

MACRONUTRIENTS

The idea behind the following sections is to add to your knowledge base so you can build awareness when putting meals together. Let's start with a closer look at macro-

nutrients—protein, carbohydrates, and fats—which are the building blocks of food. We'll kick off this conversation with protein.

Protein

While you may think of protein as coming from animal sources (meat, fish, eggs, and dairy products), plants contain protein too. Animal-based proteins contain a complete array of essential and nonessential amino acids, which are the basic components of all protein. There are nine essential amino acids, which your body can't make, so they must be supplied by the food you eat. If you eat a diet that's low in animal protein sources, it's important to combine specific plant protein sources when you eat—such as pairing rice with beans—to ensure you get all nine essential amino acids. The other eleven amino acids your body needs are nonessential, which means that while you can get them from food, your body can also make them from other amino acids.

Protein plays many roles in your body. In fact, your body uses and makes more than fifty thousand different proteins. Astonishing! It forms your muscles and helps them recover when you exercise; it is in your cell membranes and is important for cellular integrity; it forms hormones, like the blood sugar regulator insulin, and neurotransmitters, like the mood regulator serotonin. It's also found in the structural components of skin, hair, and nails, in things like collagen and keratin. The enzymes that speed up every chemical reaction in your body are made of proteins too, as are the antibodies that fight infection and the hemoglobin that carries oxygen in your blood.

Besides its role in maintaining and repairing different tissues of your body, protein is the most satiating food macronutrient and contains four calories per gram. It keeps your appetite in check, and studies have shown that it may affect whether you snack at night. People who take in less protein early in the day are more likely to snack later on—especially when willpower is low. If you've got the evening munchies, check in with your protein intake throughout the day.

Many of the women I've worked with over the years overestimate the amount of protein they actually eat. Some are afraid to eat protein because they think it will damage their kidneys or make them get bulky. A good many others simply don't realize. You don't know what you don't know! That means they miss out on protein's building blocks for recovery, satiety, hormone production, and more. If you're unsure how much

protein you're getting, now might be a good time to keep a food journal for a week to get a better picture of what you're eating.

Let's talk sourcing. The most nutrient-dense sources of protein with complete amino acid profiles are meat, fish, shellfish, eggs, and dairy products. Plant foods like nuts, seeds, legumes, beans, grains, and vegetables contain protein but in much smaller amounts. If you're a vegetarian or don't consume a lot of animal protein, be sure you're properly combining foods for a full spectrum of amino acids, and consider supplementing with crucial vitamins like B12. You may have to work a little harder to obtain adequate protein intake, especially if you're physically active. It's doable as long as you're mindful.

Before we go any further, I want to address the elephant in the room: when we think about protein, we may think only about meat, and eating meat has become more controversial in recent years. Plant-based diets are more popular than ever thanks to documentaries, social media, and even some studies that could be interpreted as concluding that meat is unhealthy. But a lot of the messaging about meat is sensationalized and divisive. It pits omnivores and herbivores against each other. In reality, we are more similar than we are different.

If my clients have reservations about eating meat, these are the points I share:

> If your body doesn't digest meat well, work with a practitioner who can help you figure out why.

> Most people could stand to eat more plants.

> Highly processed foods—animal- *and* plant-based—aren't health promoting.

> The factory farming of animals is cruel and results in lower-quality meat.

> The world would be a better place if we bought from and supported local farmers.

> Sustainability and soil health are a concern in all types of farming, including mono-crop plant agriculture.

Whether or not you eat meat is up to you, and I'm not here to force you to do anything you're not into. Take what you want and leave the rest. (Not exactly the norm when it comes to health guidance, I know . . . everyone's always arguing and pointing fingers at each other. I don't have time for that.)

The nutrition framework of the Core 4 is flexible and adaptable to your preferences. Remember that you can be paleo, gluten-free, primal, vegetarian, vegan, or whatever dietary flavor you lean toward and do it poorly. I once worked with a vegetarian whose diet consisted mostly of cheese, tortillas, coffee, and beer. Seriously, he didn't eat any vegetables! You could be paleo and eat paleo cookies all day. I know vegans who eat mostly processed food. The point is not to get super stuck on the label you slap on your eating patterns but instead to prioritize quality and what works for you. Whatever you choose, strive for a well-rounded diet with as much variety as possible, a balance of macronutrients, a full spectrum of vitamins and minerals, and plenty of fiber. If you can't get the vitamins and minerals you need because you're avoiding certain foods, it's important to supplement.

Digestion

Keep in mind that you can only assimilate and use the nutrients you can digest. Protein digestion begins in the stomach thanks to hydrochloric acid (HCl). This acid activates the enzyme pepsin, which is like a knife that chops long proteins into smaller chunks called peptides. From there, these peptides move to the small intestine, where they're further broken down by pancreatic enzymes and absorbed into the bloodstream. If you're struggling to put on muscle mass or recover after exercise despite adequate protein intake, or you feel like you can't digest protein—that is, it sits in your gut—it's worth checking with a professional to make sure all the parts of your digestive system are functioning optimally.

So how much protein do you need? It varies from person to person. The recommended daily allowance, or RDA, is often cited as the amount of protein to eat in a day. However, RDA represents a *minimum* protein intake, the quantity for basic survival, not for thriving, so I typically suggest more for my clients. Unless you're lying on the couch all day, you probably need more protein than the RDA. A good starting point for active women is 4 to 6 ounces of protein per meal, or 0.8 grams per pound of bodyweight.

Carbohydrates

Fat used to be the scary macronutrient. Luckily that's changing. Sadly, now it's carbs. Yikes! Let's take a closer look.

Carbs are a quick-burning energy source, containing four calories per gram. They're the main source of fuel for your mitochondria, the power plants in your body's cells. They're also the primary source of energy for your brain, which uses about 20 percent of your daily fuel.

Ideally, your body flexibly uses carbs and fats for energy, like a hybrid car. (Protein also can be used, but that's not a great thing for day-to-day living because it means breaking down precious muscle tissue. It could help you in a pinch, but it's far from optimal.) At any one time, your body stores about 500 grams' worth of carbs in your tissues, mostly in your muscle and a small amount in your liver. It's what you dip into during a hard workout session and at night while you sleep. Contrast that with tens of thousands of calories in stored body fat that we have hanging around at any given time. We rely on that stored energy during periods when we're at rest or when we've sapped our glycogen—stored glucose—during physical exertion.

Question: Is it better to be a sugar burner, relying on carbohydrates, or a fat burner, able to flexibly use carbs *and* fats? The modern world makes it so easy to overeat refined carbs, which causes your blood sugar to spike and then crash. (Ever feel hangry—hungry + angry? Crashing blood sugar is the culprit.) The only way to counteract the crash is to eat more carbs to prop up your energy level, because the body prefers to use glucose. Instead, let's transform you from a sugar burner, chasing the next hit of fast-acting carbs, into a fat burner with stable energy levels. Avoiding all carbs isn't necessary to become a fat burner. You'll get there by focusing on real, whole-food carb sources balanced with protein and fats.

Carbs can be either sugars or starches. The single sugars, monosaccharides, include glucose, fructose, and galactose. The disaccharides—literally double sugars—include sucrose (table sugar), lactose (milk sugar), and maltose (malt, or grain, sugar). These single and double sugars are very quickly broken down and absorbed by the body and are found in whole foods like fruits, some veggies, and sweeteners like honey and maple syrup.

Longer chains of sugars, or polysaccharides, are the starches. They store larger amounts of energy and generally take longer to digest. Nutrient-dense starches are found in foods like white potatoes, sweet potatoes, plantains, winter squashes, taro root, cassava root (yuca), rice, quinoa, legumes, and other grains.

These foods have key vitamins and minerals plus soluble fiber, which helps slow down the digestion of these foods, preventing massive blood sugar spikes. They also

contain insoluble fiber, which your body can't digest. Fiber keeps you regular, and some fibers feed your gut bacteria. These are all reasons to not be afraid of foods like apples, carrots, or sweet potatoes even though they contain "sugar."

Just like with protein, being able to digest the carbs you eat matters. Technically, you start digesting carbs in your mouth thanks to the enzyme called salivary amylase. (There's also a type of amylase that comes from your pancreas when your food is farther down the line.) If carbs hang around too long in the stomach, they can start to ferment, producing gas and making you bloated. If you're always joking about your food baby, it's probably a sign that your digestion needs support.

Once carbs leave the stomach, they're further broken down into simple sugars in your small intestine and absorbed into the bloodstream, causing blood sugar levels to rise. The pancreas releases insulin to move extra blood out of your bloodstream. It's stored for later use in your muscles and liver as a large molecule made of glucose called glycogen.

Not all carbs are created equal. When comparing them, consider how quickly each food makes your blood sugar spike and then fall. If you eat a teaspoon of table sugar (about 4 grams of carbs), your blood sugar will quickly spike and then drop. You may get a burst of energy, but it's short-lived. However, if you eat a small carrot (about 5 grams of carbs), your blood sugar won't rise as quickly. You'll get fiber, water, vitamins, and minerals along with the sugar the carrot contains, and it takes longer for your body to digest it, so your blood sugar is unlikely to soar as high and plummet so low.

While your cells can store glucose at any time, they're really good at doing it after exercise. The more muscle fibers you use during a workout, the more sensitive your body is to the signal of insulin and the easier it is to store glucose in your muscles. When you eat a chunk of carbs after a workout, your cells are better at refueling your muscle "tank" and not sending carbs to be stored away as body fat.

That's how your body *should* work. However, if you overeat carbohydrates for a long period of time, your cells may stop hearing the insulin signal, which can lead to insulin resistance.

Inflammation

Some kinds of systemic inflammation—like when you have a fever—are normal healing responses. The immune system kicks in to fight the virus or bacteria that's taking over, and then the body goes to work to stop the inflammation once you're healed. On

the other hand, chronic systemic inflammation can occur on a low-grade, body-wide level. This type of inflammation can happen because of the foods you eat, like crappy oils or too much sugar.

Often this kind of chronic systemic inflammation is rooted in your gut. If the lining of your small intestine is too porous, bits of undigested food particles get through the membrane and kick your immune system into gear. After all, the immune system recognizes substances as "you" and "not you." Those partially undigested bits of food are "not you" and shouldn't be in your bloodstream. Unlike fighting a very short-term virus, though, chronic systemic inflammation due to increased gut permeability is ongoing.

In short, chronic systemic inflammation puts a burden on your body's tissues and organs and makes you feel pretty darn crappy even though you may not realize why. It can manifest in different ways, such as fatigue; gut problems like diarrhea, constipation, and bloating; allergies; puffy eyes; brain fog; and aching joints. Insulin resistance can also contribute to this type of inflammation, which increases the risk of conditions like heart disease, type 2 diabetes, and cancer.

Get the idea? Eating an excessive amount of carbs probably isn't good for you, but you shouldn't fear them either. Eat enough carbs to support your energy needs throughout the day, and choose nourishing sources—like starchy vegetables, fruits, and gluten-free grains—as much as you can. The quality of the carbs you choose matters, so save the refined carbs and sugary treats for special occasions, if at all.

If your carb intake has been low for a while and you aren't feeling so great, you may need to tinker with it. For example, many of my clients used to eat very few carbs even though they worked out several days a week. After a while, many noticed they were tired, sluggish, and irritable, and gaining body fat around the belly. They couldn't recover from workouts and their performance wasn't what it used to be.

One possible cause is a change in thyroid function, which can occur when carbs are too low. Your body needs insulin to convert the inactive T4 hormone to the active form, T3. Going *too* low-carb can decrease your body's T3 levels. And T3 is well known for its role in controlling functions like metabolism, body temperature, and heart rate.

Eating a lower-carb diet and ditching refined sugars can help your body become more insulin sensitive (that's good!), but for some people, going too low-carb for a long period—especially if they're stressed or they work out hard—starts to produce negative effects. In other words, cutting carbs too much for too long can make it harder to feel your best.

The last piece of the carbohydrate picture is stress. Stress is going to happen. It's not "bad" per se. But it's all about the dose and recovery. Short bursts of stress followed by enough recovery are what your body is meant to handle. If a bear is chasing you, your adrenal glands release hormones like adrenaline (epinephrine), noradrenaline (norepinephrine), and cortisol. Why? You're gonna need as much energy (glucose) in your bloodstream as possible to fuel your muscles as you run like hell. Thankfully, your body has that system in place to help keep you alive. (See the sidebar "The Cortisol Connection.")

The problem is that in this modern day, longer-term stress without recovery is how many women live without even realizing it. Maybe the bear is something like your jerkface boss, money worries, undereating, the morning commute, relationship problems, toxins in your environment, or any of a host of real or perceived stressors. Your body may ramp up your blood sugar to prepare to run or fight . . . but then it doesn't happen. Often my clients see huge improvements to body composition not by continuing to push their carbs lower and lower but by dealing with their stress levels (see more about stress in the Pillar 3 chapter).

Bottom line? Include a modest amount of nourishing, whole-food carbs daily to support your energy level, workout regimen, and metabolism.

Fats

Fats are dense energy sources—they provide nine calories per gram, more than twice that of protein and carbs. And while that's fantastic in a camping situation, where you're trying to carry many calories in a small amount of space, it's easy to over-consume them in modern life. Fats are yummy, and our brains are wired to seek them out. Great when it's an avocado, maybe not when it's a monster basket of fries cooked in crappy vegetable oils and topped off with "cheez."

Though a lot of people fear fat, it's essential to your body. It's an important energy source; it forms the membranes of every one of the more than 30 trillion cells in your body; it cushions your internal organs; and it helps you absorb fat-soluble vitamins A, D, E, and K. Even cholesterol, one of the most vilified substances in history, is the precursor to many of your body's hormones, including estrogen and progesterone, two key female hormones.

The Cortisol Connection

Let's imagine our bear is back and chasing you down. It takes just fractions of a second for your brain to kick your body into gear with the fight-or-flight response. Sugar is yanked out of storage and new glucose is made, thanks to adrenaline (epinephrine), noradrenaline (norepinephrine), and cortisol.

Cortisol, in particular, is considered a master stress hormone. In addition to blood sugar, cortisol plays important roles in inflammation, blood pressure, and sleep/wake cycles. Though its jobs are necessary, when it's constantly called on due to chronic stress, things can get wacky.

Now, if there's an actual bear chasing you, great—you'll make use of that blood sugar flood, and insulin will be around after you've escaped to safety to mop up the rest. But what happens when there's no bear—no actual threat, nothing to run from, no need for a higher level of blood sugar? Over time your cells can become deaf to the signal of insulin, a state called insulin resistance. The problem isn't with these mechanisms that help keep you alive in times of threat. It's that this fight-or-flight response has been used over and over again simply to keep up with the strains of modern life—many of us live with chronic physical, emotional, and mental stress that is both real and perceived.

How do you keep cortisol in check? Eat nourishing foods. Get plenty of sleep. Work out—without overexercising. Use techniques to help you chill, something we'll talk more about in the "Get Ready" chapter.

This cortisol connection is an example of how the Core 4 pillars interrelate. You can eat a "perfect" diet as far as nutrition goes and eat an optimal amount of high-quality carbs, but if you're always feeling pressured, anxious, or under the gun, you may find it harder for you to improve your health and feel better. That interrelationship between your mind and body is one reason why it's so important to address all four pillars, together.

Your digestive system must be able to break down and absorb the fats you eat as it does protein and carbs. Your gallbladder plays an important role in this process, releasing bile to emulsify the fats you've eaten and get them ready for absorption. The pancreas gets involved too, sending special enzymes that break down fats. Essential fatty acid

deficiency is common among my clients, even when they appear to be eating enough. When they start supporting their liver and gallbladder, fat digestion often improves. One way to tell whether you're digesting fats well is to check out your poop. Seriously. A little gross? Nah. It'll tell you a lot about your gut health. If it's greasy and leaves an oily slick in the bowl, something may not be right with fat digestion.

Fats are primarily made of fatty acid chains of varying lengths and are grouped into two families: saturated and unsaturated. Saturated fats generally come from animal sources, for example, butter, lard, tallow, and duck fat, with the notable exceptions of coconut and palm kernel oils, plant-based fats that contain a higher percentage of saturated fat. Unsaturated fats include canola, olive, safflower, and sesame oils. Nuts and seeds also contain unsaturated fat.

Let's get science-y for a moment and explore how these fats differ. Saturated fats have long chains of single-bonded fatty acids. They lie straight and cluster close together like a bunch of straws. Since they pack so closely together, they're usually solid at room temperature. Unsaturated fats, however, have some double bonds in their chains, and wherever there is a double bond, the chain bends. Imagine a pile of bendy straws. Monounsaturated fats ("mono" means "one") have one bend in the chain. Polyunsaturated fats ("poly" means "many") have more than one bend in the chain. That's why these fats are usually liquid at room temperature. The more bends, or kinks, in the chain the fatty acid has, the more fragile and "breakable" it tends to be.

Monounsaturated fats are more stable than their polyunsaturated cousins. When the latter is exposed to heat or light, they tend to break down or oxidize and release cell-damaging free radicals. Think of free radicals as bad guys that float around the body—they're formed when oxygen interacts with certain atoms or molecules, making them negatively charged and looking for trouble. Free radicals are problematic because they can cause chain reactions that damage important cellular bits like DNA. Left unchecked, free radicals can cause disease and accelerate aging. Luckily, antioxidants—like the ones found in veggies and fruit—are like the cops that stop free-radical baddies in their tracks. Another reason to eat your broccoli!

We're still dealing with fat phobia from the last few decades of the twentieth century. So many of the women I work with still avoid egg yolks, swap out butter for margarine, and opt for nonfat dairy products. Let's all take a moment of silence for the death of flavor, satisfaction, and health benefits. Like a game of Telephone, the message continues

Omega-3 and Omega-6 Fatty Acids

There are two special classes of polyunsaturated fatty acids: linoleic acid (LA), also called omega-6 fatty acid, and alpha-linolenic acid (ALA), also called omega-3 fatty acid. Eicosapentaenoic acid (EPA) and docosahexaenoic acid (DHA) are two types of omega-3 fatty acids well known for their anti-inflammatory effect in the body. Though omega-6 fatty acids play an important role in the inflammatory process, a significant *imbalance* between them and omega-3 fatty acids is thought to be a growing problem.

Inflammation isn't bad per se. If you get a cut, your body mounts a rapid inflammatory response to help the area heal. It gets red and hot from increased blood flow, and you might even notice some swelling. Your immune system kicks in to prevent infection. Cool, right? We need this acute inflammatory response to heal. On the other hand, long-term, low-grade inflammation sucks. This type of system-wide inflammation may go on for weeks, months, or possibly years. There's evidence that this type of inflammation puts you at higher risk for chronic disease.

Both omega-3 and omega-6 are *essential* fatty acids, which means—as it does with amino acids—that your body can't make them, so you have to get them through food.

Rich food sources of omega-3s include salmon, sardines, and other fatty, cold-water fish; grass-fed meats; ground flaxseed or cold-pressed flax oil; chia seeds; nuts like walnuts and pecans; and egg yolks. Omega-6 fatty acids can be found in plant oils, such as the oils of peanuts, black currant seeds, evening primrose seeds, and borage seeds, plus in some meats, but—and this is a big but—the bulk of omega-6s in the modern diet come from crappy industrial seed oils that are often degraded and oxidized by the time they are consumed. Because these cheap, low-quality oils—such as corn, cottonseed, safflower, sunflower, and soybean—are ubiquitous in packaged and processed foods, it's easy to overdo it.

Including some omega-6 in your diet is important because it does have benefits, such as supporting bone health and helping with the inflammatory process, but be mindful of the source. In our modern diet, the current ratio of omega-6s to omega-3s is somewhere in the neighborhood of forty to one, hugely unbalanced; instead, it should be between one to one and four to one. Avoiding processed foods and industrial seed oils is the simplest way to reduce your omega-6 intake and get your ratio within a better range.

to get twisted, leaving the average consumer confused and unsure. Consider this: even the US government—(in)famous for advocating low-fat diets—changed its stance on dietary cholesterol in 2016, calling it no longer "a nutrient of concern."

But the damage is done and there's still a lot of fear about eating animal fats, which are saturated and contain cholesterol, with people opting instead for cheaper unsaturated vegetable oils like corn, canola, sunflower, and soybean. However, not only is much of the concern about saturated fat overblown and frankly unfounded, unsaturated fats aren't completely innocent. They're far more fragile than saturated fats, which means they break down easily, especially during high-temperature cooking and even during the process of oil extraction itself. When they break down, they release free radicals. So when you opt for french fries cooked in highly processed, oxidized oil that has been heated and reheated for days, that "heart-healthy" unsaturated fat loses its luster!

You don't have to avoid fried foods forever, but you'll want to limit these cheap oils and aim for a *combination* of healthy saturated and unsaturated fats from a variety of sources. Stick to real, whole-food sources of fats and oils from high-quality, cold-pressed, and grass-fed sources. Mix a variety of animal and plant fats into your routine, but don't go nuts (no pun intended). That means half a jar of almond butter isn't a snack. My favorite fat sources are grass-fed butter and ghee, coconut products, olives, nuts, and seeds. (See the Nourishing Foods Framework coming up soon, on pages 34–35.)

MICRONUTRIENTS

Eating a variety of different proteins, carbohydrates, and fats—macronutrients—makes it more likely you'll also get a wide spectrum of micronutrients, vitamins and minerals. It can be convenient to prepare the same dishes all the time, but that's a surefire way to end up lacking in certain nutrients. Make it fun: trying one new fruit or veggie each week is a good way to break out of a food rut.

Vitamins

Our bodies can't make most vitamins, which assist with hundreds of important functions, so we have to get them from our food or take supplements. Fortunately, nutrient-

dense real foods have vitamins packaged together in the way nature intended—many work in conjunction with other vitamins, vitamin cofactors, and minerals.

Vitamins are either fat-soluble or water-soluble. Fat-soluble vitamins include A, D, E, and K and are found in full-fat dairy, meat, organ meat, fish, eggs, nuts, seeds, and dark leafy greens. As the name implies, they're stored in our fat tissue. Water-soluble vitamins include the B vitamins and C, and they are found in vegetables, fruits, legumes, nuts, seeds, whole grains, egg yolks, dairy, meat, organ meat, and fish. These vitamins are water soluble, so you must have a fairly regular supply through your diet. A note about vitamin B12: it's found in sufficient amounts only in animal products (meat, organ meat, fish, eggs), so vegans may need to supplement.

Minerals

We must get minerals, like vitamins, from what we eat. They play many different roles in our health, including helping muscle contraction and nerve impulses, moving substances across cell membranes, assisting as coenzymes, and maintaining bone structure. You've probably heard of calcium, magnesium, sodium, potassium, iron, zinc, and iodine—but there are many more.

One of the most commonly deficient minerals in the body is magnesium—it's estimated that nearly half of adults don't get enough. Lack of this mineral may affect everything from how well your cells produce energy to the strength of your immune system and even your food cravings. In fact, if you crave chocolate, you may be low in magnesium! Other magnesium-rich foods include dark leafy greens, avocados, nuts, and seeds.

FERMENTED FOODS

Beyond all the rich macro- and micronutrients the recipes in this program will provide, your body will also benefit from fermented foods. These have been part of human food preservation for thousands of years and are well loved by cultures all around the world. They typically contain probiotic bacteria to help support the gut, and since they're raw, they contain beneficial enzymes and acids.

Since incorporating fermented foods into my daily routine years ago, I have seen huge improvements in my digestion, skin quality, and immunity, just to name a few.

It's estimated that 70 to 80 percent of your immune system is in your gut, so supporting it with the right flora helps keep everything working correctly. I started by making my own sauerkraut and branched out into drinks like kombucha and beet kvass in addition to kimchi and other fermented veggies.

Sometimes I buy my fermented foods—there's nothing wrong with that if you're too busy! You'll want to look for products that are refrigerated and raw, not pasteurized. Aim for a couple of forkfuls of fermented veggies with breakfast or about 4 ounces of a fermented beverage like kombucha or water kefir, to start.

NOURISHING FOODS FRAMEWORK: AN OVERVIEW

The foods you'll eat during the Core 4 program will make you feel more energized, clear minded, and stronger. Along with needed macronutrients, they contain lots of vitamins, minerals, soluble and insoluble fiber, and antioxidants. They're also minimally processed, colorful, and encourage stable blood sugar levels.

A clear framework may make it easier for you to get started, but remember that no two people will settle on the same exact mix of foods that makes them feel their best. For a quick reference chart, see the Nourishing Foods Framework on pages 34–35.

Tier 1 Foods

Tier 1 foods are your go-tos, the foods you'll focus on adding to your routine. They're dense in nutrients and naturally make you feel full and content. In other words, these foods contain a combination of calories, macronutrients, and satiety factors that tell your brain to stop eating when your body has had enough. For the duration of the 30-day Core 4 program, you'll be focusing mostly on Tier 1 foods.

Note that if you know a Tier 1 food doesn't work for your body, you should leave it out or make a substitution.

Tier 1 foods are

- meat, seafood, and eggs for protein;
- veggies, fruits, and good-for-you starches, like winter squashes and sweet potatoes, for carbohydrates;
- healthy fats and oils, like avocado, butter (yes, butter!), coconut oil, and olive oil; and

- fermented veggies and bone broth as boosters. (Bone broth is rich in collagen—your grandma was on to something!)

Shopping for Tier 1 Foods

You can find the vast majority of the ingredients you'll need during the program in a regular supermarket, natural grocer, or local supplier. If you can't, check with an online retailer like Thrive Market. Since these foods are your nutritional powerhouses, try to include protein, carbs, and healthy fats at each meal for a wide array of macronutrients, micronutrients, antioxidants, and fiber.

For proteins, opt for grass-fed, pastured, free-range, and/or organic options when you can. These options may not always be available or in your budget, and some of these labels can mean vastly different things. However, higher-quality proteins typically contain more nutrients and in many cases mean the animals had a better quality of life. If that's out of budget, trim or drain excess fat off the meat you buy, or opt for leaner meats. If you can, get to know a local organic farmer or rancher.

For the veggies and fruits, aim for organic, seasonal, and/or locally grown when possible. Produce in season is more affordable (it's all about supply and demand!), and local produce is typically fresher and therefore higher in nutrients. Buying local produce also supports the economy in your area and cuts down on transportation time—those strawberries you buy in January probably got to you via airplane or long-distance trucking. If organic isn't in your budget, consult the Environmental Working Group's Dirty Dozen, the Shopper's Guide to Pesticide in Produce (EWG.org /foodnews/dirty-dozen.php), to prioritize your dollars.

For fats and oils, opt for high-quality animal fats from pastured and/or grass-fed animals and cold-pressed oils. Better-quality animal fats will be richer in nutrients. Cold-pressed plant oils aren't produced with gnarly chemicals or heat, which can damage the more fragile unsaturated fats.

Tier 2 Foods

After the 30-day Core 4 program, you may want to experiment with these foods and see how they affect your body. Though I've included a few Tier 2 foods in the recipes you'll find later in the book, remember that your bioindividuality—your current health status

and genetics—means certain foods may work for you while others won't. These foods, though nutrient-dense and staples of many cultures, may cause digestive problems, skin irritation, joint inflammation, and other issues in some people. In other people, these foods are tolerated just fine. It may be worth doing a short elimination to gather some observations. On the other hand, you may already know that some of these foods work well for you because you've experimented before. In that case, feel free to include them right away. Some whole grains are included in this group, and I recommend sticking to unrefined, gluten-free whole grains most of the time. Many of my clients feel better when they avoid gluten-containing whole grains such as wheat, barley, and rye, as well as gluten-containing refined-grain products like most pasta and bread, so I've left those out of the framework. If you're unsure, follow the recommended framework for thirty days and see how you feel. Just because a food is gluten-free doesn't mean it's minimally processed or good for your blood sugar! Some gluten-free packaged foods may cause blood sugar to spike more than their gluten-filled counterparts.

Note any negative changes in your energy level, mood, and digestion if you include these foods. You may decide to further experiment with a food, keep a food journal, or talk to your health-care provider for more guidance.

Tier 2 foods are

- full-fat dairy products, like milk, cheese, yogurt, and cream;
- properly soaked and sprouted whole grains and grain-like foods, like rice, quinoa, and oats;
- properly soaked and sprouted legumes, like beans and lentils;
- unrefined sweeteners, like honey and maple syrup (they're still sugar so you'll want to use them judiciously); and
- alcohol.

Shopping for Tier 2 Foods

If during the Core 4 program you decide to remove even the few Tier 2 foods I've included in the recipes and afterward you'd like to reintroduce them, do so by adding one category at a time for three days, and note any differences. Remember, the goal is

What About Alcohol?

Wondering about alcohol? Alcohol contains 7 calories per gram, and the wine, beer, or spirits you may enjoy contain primarily carbs. And despite what people may say, no one's really drinking wine for the antioxidants—am I right?!

So let's talk about this straight. Some people can easily moderate alcohol with no issues. Others don't like how they feel after drinking, or they use alcohol to unwind or fall asleep (which causes a whole host of problems we'll discuss in the Pillar 4 chapter), or it opens the gateway to poor food choices.

If that sounds like you, I recommend you try some of the habit-change work you'll learn about in the "Get Ready" chapter. And if you feel adamant you will *fight anyone who tries to take away your wine,* maybe that's a sign something deeper is going on.

Also, I suggest taking a break if you're aiming for body recomposition (alcohol is high in calories with low nutritive value), if you're in perimenopause or menopause (the body has a harder time processing alcohol), or you have sleep problems (alcohol is a sleep disruptor). At the end of the day, if you suspect alcohol isn't working for you, remove it for a month and see what happens. Sparkling flavored water and herbal tea are my two favorite alcohol substitutes.

to include as wide a variety of real, whole, properly prepared, nutrient-dense foods in your routine as possible!

Tier 3 Foods

Finally, let's look at the Tier 3 foods, the ones to minimize, both during the Core 4 program and in the future. These foods don't have a place in a daily nourishing dietary routine and are the opposite of health promoting. They're highly refined and stripped of their vitamins, minerals, and fiber. In fact, vitamins and minerals may be added back in afterward in an attempt to make these foods appear healthier than they are. Some of these foods spawn free radicals that damage cells, and others totally whack out your blood sugar. Nobody's perfect, though! If you do eat these foods from time to

time, make the next meal better and move on. No need to punish yourself or play the "I'll start again on Monday" game.

Tier 3 foods are

- refined grain products (including refined corn and rice products, plus barley, rye, wheat, etc.);

- processed soy, unless it's been traditionally fermented;

- refined and artificial sugars;

- industrial vegetable oils (corn, canola, cottonseed, grapeseed, peanut, safflower, soybean, sunflower, etc.); and

- hydrogenated oils and other trans fats (margarine and other butter substitutes).

At least for the duration of the Core 4 program, I highly recommend you eliminate these foods and see how you feel.

General Eating Guidelines for the Program (and Beyond)

If your eating schedule is erratic or inconsistent, try switching to a regular schedule. You'll be more satiated and experience fewer cravings. Over time, as you start listening to your body and eating more intuitively, you may discover you do better with two big meals and a snack, four smaller meals, of some other combination. Customizing for your own needs and preferences takes experimentation. If you're not sure how to start, begin with three meals to establish a routine and go from there. Get comfortable with the basics before you try anything fancy.

If you're still hungry after a meal, have a small snack with protein, carbs, and fat to tide you over till the next meal.

If you're constantly hungry, slowly increase the amount of protein and/or fat at each meal.

Relax before you eat. Chew your food and eat with as few distractions as possible.

Aim to feel comfortably full, not stuffed. It takes a while for your brain to get the signal that your stomach is full.

THE BATTLE AGAINST YOUR ENVIRONMENT

Now that you have a better understanding of all the goodness in the nutrient-dense foods you'll soon be eating on this program, let's consider why it's so challenging to eat enough of these foods each day.

Nutrient-dense foods are sort of self-limiting in the amount you can eat. Imagine sitting down to a juicy chicken breast. The first few bites taste insanely good, but you start to get filled up quickly. By the time you're halfway through your chicken, it's not as exciting as it was at the start. Foods like sweet potatoes or salmon or carrots or quinoa fill you up faster because of their protein, fiber, and nutrient content. On the other hand, how easy is it to polish off an entire bag of chips in one sitting?

Our modern environment sets us up for challenges. We're surrounded by a plethora of easily available, very yummy foods that are engineered to taste better than anything found in nature. When these sugary, fatty, salty, crunchy foods ping your brain's reward center, you typically choose the path of least resistance. That's just human nature. It's not just you. You're not crazy or weak or lacking willpower. Couple that with how easy it is to be sedentary and stressed, and you've got quite the situation on your hands.

But giving in doesn't have to be your fate. The Core 4 will be your guide with simple—though let's be real, not always easy—changes that make it possible to navigate this tricky modern life. Making better choices, being consistent, and going against the grain is key. Just because everyone else is doing it doesn't make it right. So fly that little revolutionary flag because you're winning the battle with this program.

When you start adding more nourishing foods to your routine, you'll find it easier to crowd out food that doesn't make you feel as good. Just remember, dialing in your unique best nutrition doesn't only mean adding things. You're also taking care to avoid those nutrient-poor, inflammatory, craving-inducing Tier 3 foods because you're putting most of your attention on all the tasty, nourishing, satisfying foods *you get to eat*. Same end result, different mindset.

Nourishing Foods Framework

TIER 1 NOURISHING FOODS ⟵————————————➤

These are your nutritional powerhouses. Include protein, carbs, and healthy fats at each meal for a full spectrum of macronutrients, vitamins, minerals, antioxidants, and fiber.

Proteins

Aim for grass-fed, pastured, free-range, and/or organic whenever possible

Beef
Bison
Chicken
Duck
Eggs
Elk
Fish
Lamb
Organ meats
Pork
Seafood
Shellfish
Turkey
Venison

Carbs: Veggies

Aim for organic, in season, and/or local whenever possible

Artichokes
Arugula
Asparagus
Bok choy
Brussels
  sprouts
Cabbage
Carrots
Cauliflower
Celery
Collard greens
Cucumber
Eggplant
Garlic
Green beans
Green onions
Jicama
Kale
Leeks
Lettuces
Mushrooms
Onions
Peppers
Radishes
Snap or snow
  peas
Spaghetti
  squash
Spinach
Sprouts
Summer
  squash
Swiss chard
Tomatoes
Turnips
Zucchini

Carbs: Starchy Veggies

Aim for organic, in season, and/or local whenever possible

Beets
Cassava root
  (or yuca)
Lotus root
Parsnips
Plantains
Rutabagas
Sweet
  potatoes
Taro root
White potatoes
Winter squash
  (acorn,
  delicata,
  butternut,
  kabocha,
  pumpkin,
  spaghetti,
  etc.)
Yams

Carbs: Fruit

Aim for organic, in season, and/or local whenever possible

Apples
Apricots
Bananas
Blackberries
Blueberries
Cherries
Grapefruits
Grapes
Kiwifruits
Lemons
Limes
Mangoes
Nectarines
Oranges
Papayas
Peaches
Pears
Pineapples
Plums
Pomegranates
Raspberries
Watermelons

Fats and Oils

Aim for high-quality fats from pastured/grass-fed animals and cold-pressed oils

Avocados and
  avocado oil
Bacon and
  bacon fat
Butter
Coconut
  flakes, milk,
  and oil
Duck fat
Egg yolks
Ghee (clarified
  butter)
Lard
Nuts
  (almonds,
  Brazil nuts,
  cashews,
  hazelnuts,
  walnuts, etc.)
Olives and
  olive oil
Red palm oil
Seeds
  (chia, flax,
  pumpkin,
  sesame,
  sunflower,
  etc.)
Tallow

Fermented Foods and Nourishment Boosters

Aim for high-quality store-bought or homemade

Bone broth
Kimchi
Kombucha
Kvass
Pickled
  veggies (low
  sugar)
Sauerkraut
  (raw)
Water kefir
. . . and
  any other
  fermented
  veggies (raw)

TIER 2 TEST-IT-OUT FOODS ←——————————→

These are foods I highly recommend you eliminate for a month and see how you feel. They may cause sensitivities, allergies, and inflammation in many people. Afterward, if you'd like to reintroduce them, do so by adding one category at a time for three days. Note any differences.

Dairy
Full-fat, pastured/ grass-fed, raw, and/ or organic

Cheese
Cream
Milk
Yogurt

Legumes
Properly soaked and sprouted

Beans
Lentils

Gluten-free Whole Grains
Properly soaked and sprouted

Buckwheat
Corn
Gluten-free oats
Quinoa
Rice

Natural Sweeteners
Honey (raw and locally sourced)
Maple syrup

Alcohol
Beer
Cider
Gluten-free beer
Liquor
Spirits
Wine

TIER 3 AVOID-WHEN-POSSIBLE FOODS ←——————————→

These are foods I highly recommend you eliminate for a month and see how you feel. They may cause sensitivities, allergies, and inflammation in many people.

Hydrogenated fats (margarine and other butter substitutes)
Refined grains (refined rice or corn products, etc.)
Refined sugars
Soy (unless traditionally fermented)

Trans fats
Vegetable oils (corn, canola, cottonseed, grapeseed, safflower, soybean, sunflower, etc.)

Note About Portions

Inevitably, any conversation about nourishing foods eventually turns to portion size. A seven-day food journal and/or food tracking with an app may help you get a handle on portions, especially since it's quite common to have portion distortion. However, if you have a history of disordered eating, exercise caution when logging or tracking food and consult a professional.

Instead of long-term tracking, I recommend a visual system. You may have to adjust this baseline depending on your body size and activity level, but here is a guide to eyeballing a single portion size per meal:

Avocado: ¼ to ½ of an avocado

Eggs: 2 to 4

Fermented drinks like kombucha or kefir: 4 to 8 ounces a day

Fermented veggies: a generous forkful

Fruits, starchy veggies, gluten-free grains, and legumes: 1 to 1.5 cupped open hand(s)

Meats and fish: palm-to-hand sized

Nuts, seeds, animal fats, and oils: 1 to 2 thumb-sized portions

Vegetables: 2+ cupped open hands . . . aim for at least half the plate

Satiety and Satiation

While we're on the subject, let's talk about the difference between satiety and satiation, which are two related but different concepts. Satiation is the more immediate feeling of fullness that occurs when you eat. Satiety, however, is the longer-term experience after eating—how long your hunger is satisfied.

Satiety is affected by how much fiber and protein is in food, for example. Satiety is complex and spans the time from when you put food into your mouth until long after its digested nutrients have been absorbed. One interesting way food affects satiety is by its texture; that is, liquid foods have a weaker effect on satiety than solids, which need to be chewed. That's one of the reasons why I recommend limiting shakes, blended coffee drinks, and other calorie-dense, but lower satiety, liquids if you're trying to improve your health.

When it comes to regulating appetite, the two main hunger hormones are leptin and ghrelin. Leptin is made by your fat cells. Higher leptin tells the body, "We have enough stored energy here," so if you have adequate stores of body fat, it ratchets down your appetite. Ghrelin, made by the stomach when it's empty, signals when it's time to eat and returns to its baseline after you've had a meal. When you're dieting and really cutting calories, the cruel irony is that ghrelin spikes, causing you to seek out food. This is why I don't recommend drastic caloric restriction as a long-term weight-loss strategy.

When they work properly, leptin and ghrelin do a pretty good job of regulating appetite. But in recent years, there has been more research into whether these messengers work properly in some people. Is it possible that your cells can't "hear" the leptin signal, for example, making you feel insatiably hungry? Hopefully more research will provide answers. One thing is clear: the regulation of appetite is complex. But when you eat high-satiety nutrient-dense foods, don't overly restrict calories, build muscle, and get more sleep, you can make progress. And the nourishing foods you'll eat on the Core 4 will keep you satiated.

BEYOND THE "WHAT" OF NUTRITION

Eating nourishing foods is about *what* you eat. But *how* and *when* you eat are just as important. And that requires becoming more mindful—paying attention to your eat-

ing habits. As a society, we're hyper-distracted and multitasking our faces off. We scroll social media while we eat. (My biggest challenge.) We eat in our cars, at our desks, in front of the TV. We're often in a stressed-out state. We sit down with friends and loved ones less and less . . . the concept of gathering around a table to share nourishing food and conversation is all but disappearing. And we skip meals or try to graze every two hours to keep blood sugar from crashing and burning. All of this results in poor digestion, undernutrition, blood sugar problems, and disconnection—from each other and from our food.

Eating has been reduced to a chore instead of an occasion to connect with one another and with the food we've taken the time to prepare. When was the last time you sat down and tried to savor the taste of what you were eating? How you eat is important for more than just satiety. Your body has two branches—the sympathetic and the parasympathetic—within the autonomic nervous system, and they operate almost like yin and yang. The sympathetic arm is responsible for the fight-or-flight response when you're stressed or threatened. Even low-level, everyday stressors, like someone cutting you off in traffic, can kick the sympathetic nervous system into high gear, and eating when you're in that heightened state makes digestion more difficult.

Think of this from a threat point of view. If our bear popped out of the woods while you were hiking, your sympathetic nervous system would really kick in. Your heart rate and respiration would increase, thanks to adrenaline and noradrenaline. Blood would be diverted away from your internal organs to your arms and legs so you could fight or flee. That's not an optimal situation in which to eat and digest food—your body isn't primed to do it.

The parasympathetic system is the opposite: it's the rest-and-digest part that takes over when you're relaxed. You want the parasympathetic system at work when you're eating. Yet most of us often eat on the go, when we're distracted and stressed, which prevents the body from chilling out during mealtime. When you learn to eat mindfully, your body is better able to digest and assimilate the nutrients in the food you eat.

Turning on the Parasympathetic System

So how do you slide your system from sympathetic to parasympathetic at meal time? We've become so disconnected from what we're eating. We don't typically grow the

food we eat; often we don't even cook it ourselves. Food has become something we just shove into our mouths without thinking about it.

To turn on your parasympathetic system, you can start with something as simple as taking a few deep breaths and expressing gratitude for your food. Treat mealtime as its own occasion, not a nuisance. Bring attention to what you're eating, whether that's turning off your electronic devices or taking time to smell, savor, and enjoy your food.

When you eat while you're doing something else, you're not focusing on the flavors, textures, or satisfaction of the food. When your mind is distracted, you're not associating eating with anything else—not with gratitude for the food itself or for the person who prepared it for you or even for the opportunity to nourish your body.

Yes, you're busy and stressed and probably in a rush. But when you eat without slowing down and being mindful about what you're eating, the process becomes a robotic task with little pleasure. Hey, I do this sometimes myself! I'm not perfect! But when you eat mindfully, you give your mind and body a much-needed break from the demands of your day.

Take these steps to eat more mindfully and engage your parasympathetic system:

SIT DOWN. Yes, start simple. And that means sitting at the dining table or, if you must, your desk—not behind the wheel of your car. (Eating and driving is a terrible combination. You're distracted by your food as you drive and distracted by driving as you eat.) Take a couple of deep breaths and bring your attention to what you're going to eat. You may want to think or say something you're grateful for. Bonus points for sitting on the floor. There's something so grounding about eating from that position.

TURN OFF YOUR ELECTRONICS. Remove all distractions, whether it's television or social media. Start looking at eating as an opportunity to slow down and take a break.

USE YOUR SENSES. As the saying goes, you eat with your eyes first. How does the food look? How appealing is it? How does it smell? Is your mouth watering already? Anticipating what you're about to eat makes the experience more pleasurable and jump-starts your digestive system.

TAKE SMALL BITES. Your mom was right—don't wolf down your food. Smaller bites slow your pace and let you savor what you're eating. Put your fork down between bites. Take small sips of water. Whatever slows down your eating.

CHEW WELL. Chewing is the start of mechanical digestion. The process of chewing tells your body, "Get ready to receive nutrients!" And as you saw a few pages ago, chewing introduces digestive enzymes into the mix and improves satiety.

INVITE SOMEONE TO JOIN YOU. When you eat with someone else, you increase your sense of community and connection. Sharing a meal or simply eating with a coworker can help you feel less isolated.

EATING ON THE GO: SIMPLE HACKS TO MAKE THE BEST CHOICES

It's easier to choose nutritious foods when you're eating at home—especially after you learn how to prepare meals in advance. But what about when you're on the go? Use these simple hacks to make smart choices away from home.

AVOID FOOD WITH LABELS WHEN POSSIBLE. Whole, natural, nutritious foods usually come without labels—and you're almost always better off choosing a food like this over a processed one. If you're stuck and have to buy something prepackaged, choose an item that has fewer ingredients than more.

SHOP SMART. If you have time to grab something at the grocery store, stick to the outside edges of the market—that's where you'll find the fresh food sections. Processed and packaged foods are found in the aisles.

READ CAREFULLY. Eating out? Look for foods that are baked, roasted, steamed, or poached, and skip those that are fried, deep-fried, breaded, or "crispy." Fried restaurant foods are cooked in low-quality vegetable oils that have been heated over and over again. Ask for oil and vinegar instead of dressings with dodgy oils, and request that condiments like mayonnaise be served on the side so you can control how much is added. If a dish is served with sauce, ask whether it has been thickened with flour if you're sensitive to gluten.

ASK FOR SUBSTITUTIONS. Ask your server if you can swap something else in—a side salad or vegetable instead of a side of fries, for example. If you're ordering an entrée salad, ask how much protein comes with it. I've ordered salads that came with only two dinky strips of chicken on top, and I was hungry an hour later. Ask to double the protein on the salad, swap in nuts or seeds for croutons, or add a hard-boiled egg or two, and leave off the cheese if dairy is an issue for you.

SNACK SMARTER. Whether you're eating a meal or a snack, try to combine the three macronutrients—protein, carbs, and healthy fats—for better blood sugar control and satiety. Even at a quickie mart, you can probably find, say, a banana and some beef jerky—whole foods that keep you going for hours.

PLAN AHEAD. Having a go-to snack in your purse or bag can be a lifesaver when you're hungry. Hard-boiled eggs, unsalted almonds, grain-free granola, jerky, dehydrated fruit chips, kale chips, veggies and hummus, and fresh fruit all make great portable snacks.

KEEP IT SIMPLE

Let me add one more thing here. As I mentioned at the beginning of this chapter, the problem with complex nutrition rules and super-restrictive diets is that they aren't sustainable. The harder and more limiting a diet is, the less likely you are to stick to it . . . and that's the enemy of consistency, the thing that helps you gain health.

Also, trying to make a fifteen-step healthy recipe you found on Pinterest on a frantically busy Tuesday night will leave you feeling stressed and resentful—not exactly the way to make progress. Stick with the basics, stay consistent over time, and watch how you start to look and feel better without all the hassle and heartbreak of diets.

In the next chapter, we'll switch gears from what you feed your body to how you move it, in the second of the Core 4 pillars, "Move with Intention."

Move with Intention

Exercise. The word is enough to make you wrinkle your nose in disgust. Somewhere along the way, you were probably convinced that you have to suffer through exercise you hate in order to see results. I'm here to change all that. I'm going to show you how to strengthen your body and boost your confidence while also enjoying the process, and you'll get better results in less time.

I know, building strength totally fucks with the narrative we have always been taught: that women can't—or shouldn't—be strong. That we should be tiny. And stay small. And take up less space. And shrink to make others feel comfortable. There are endless layers—racism, classism, ableism, sexism, and ageism—beneath these concepts. For many women I work with, building physical strength and taking up more space aren't just ways to express their individuality and values; they're acts of unapologetic resistance. No matter what this means to you, simply by engaging with the Core 4 and this pillar, you'll do things differently from what society may expect.

Moving with intention doesn't mean just lifting weights. (And trust me, this goes beyond tiny pink dumbbells.) Oh no. It's so much more than that. I want you to expand your view and think about a strong body in much broader terms. Moving in ways that honor this wondrous body you were gifted instead of punishing it might be a strategy

you're not used to. Coming to a place where you trust and respect your body—and you're able to listen to your intuition—may take effort, but it's not impossible.

The Core 4 framework for strengthening your body is to

move your body intentionally—every day;

strength train with total-body compound movements a few times a week;

sprinkle in some interval-based cardio as your health and schedule allow or do other activities you love; and

perform routine maintenance on yourself.

With consistency, you'll improve your strength, coordination, mobility, flexibility, balance, power, and endurance—all important factors in being a more resilient, unbreakable human. A capable, healthy, balanced body will take you far.

MUSCLE MATTERS: THE KEY TO THE STRENGTH PILLAR

Let's face it, women and muscle haven't always been a popular combination. There's a fear of getting bulky and looking like the Incredible Hulk. And when muscle building *is* discussed, the terms "long and lean" and "toned" get tossed around. So first things first: you cannot make your muscles longer; that's 100 percent genetic. When women say they want to be "toned," that means adding muscle definition. That's achieved by strength training coupled with good nutrition choices and plenty of sleep. There's no such thing as spot toning.

What if you don't love strength training? What if you're scared to try it? The most important thing to take away from this chapter is to commit to the kind of movement you *love*, because that way you'll actually do it, be consistent, and see results. It should bring you joy and satisfaction. The power of strength training is real, and I've seen so many women flourish when they start moving with weights. So my mission is to combine the two for you: to teach you how to strength train and to help you fall in love with it so you'll make it a regular part of your life. Here's the thing: there are many ways to move your body with intention, to show

it care and respect, and to help it get stronger. If you want to experience the most efficient—and in my experience, the most powerful—way to get stronger and live bigger in so many ways, I've got the framework that can help. And it's so much simpler than you think.

The fastest, most efficient way to build muscle is with total-body movements that work major muscle groups and smaller stabilizing muscles. Use it all, woman! And you have to use your muscles regularly to maintain them. Remember, though, that our modern environment is working against you when it comes to moving and strengthening your body. It's so easy to opt out of movement, even when it comes to the most mundane tasks. But this isn't just about asking little Bobby down the street to mow your lawn once a week. You may sit nearly all day at work. Even in our leisure time, we all sit more than we used to.

We evolved from roaming hunter-gatherers to mostly agricultural societies. And though that shift took place thousands of years ago, being active is still coded in our DNA. Undoubtedly, our hunter-gatherer ancestors didn't have to swing by the gym in the afternoon because a higher baseline of movement was built into their daily activities.

As modern humans, we're experiencing the opposite. You've probably got to go out of your way to be active. Gyms are relatively new inventions, places for us to deliberately move outside home or work. Plus, now you can pay someone to do literally almost anything for you. You don't have to plant, tend, harvest, prepare, or even cook your own food any longer. Food apps make it possible to have your meals delivered right to your door. They show up ready to eat. All you have to do is chew. (Nobody's developed a way to outsource that . . . yet.) That's just one example of how easy it is to move less and less. **You have to consciously create opportunities to pick up some heavy shit, to move around more, and to take care of yourself.**

As a culture that's obsessed with being "not fat," we're missing the real star of the show: muscle. Muscle mass is a better predictor of longevity than fat mass. Muscle provides protection against disease and illness, serving as an extra reserve when times are tough. It powers your movement, whether that's climbing up a ladder to clean your gutters, keeping up with your kids, or hauling a load of wet laundry from the washing machine to the dryer.

Once you're in your thirties, you begin to lose muscle. You've got to maintain what you do have and build more to turn the ship around. The way to do that is by "progressive overload." That's a fancy term for gradually lifting heavier weights, which causes your muscles to adapt.

You don't have to be *extreme* to get stronger. Constantly nudging your body—challenging it a little bit at a time—is a smarter way to work. After a strength-training session, your body repairs any microdamage to the muscle tissue. The result is denser, stronger muscle (but not necessarily larger—see the sidebar "Bulky, Schmulky!" on page 49). You get stronger during recovery, not during the workout itself.

As your body's natural healing ability performs the tissue repair, it's aided by what you eat. Eating enough protein to repair muscle is essential. Muscle recovery takes place on a longer timeline than you might think—it may take a week or more to completely recover from a heavy deadlift. Some people think the window for post-workout recovery slams shut thirty minutes after a workout, but that's misguided. Your body will be more insulin sensitive closer to finishing your workout, so it's easier to shuttle nutrients back into your cells. Since muscle recovery takes place on a longer timeline, eating a variety of nourishing foods in your daily routine matters.

If you miss the thirty-minute window, it's not the end of the world. But if you're not recovering well, try getting some protein and carbs sooner after you finish your workout. Signs of poor recovery include things like lingering stiffness or soreness, loss of power or strength, an overall decline in performance, disruptions in mood and/or sleep, and even getting sick a lot.

In short, the most efficient ways to build muscle are the following:

Lift weights that place appropriately challenging demands on your muscles.

Prioritize compound, multi-joint movements. (For example, a shoulder press uses more muscles than a biceps curl.)

Try eating a post-workout meal of 20 to 30 grams of protein and 40 to 60 grams of carbs within thirty minutes of working out if you train hard on consecutive days.

Take enough time off, using active and passive recovery techniques, and treat your body well. Recovery matters!

A QUICK LOOK AT THE CORE 4 WORKOUTS

The Core 4 workouts give you an option to choose from two workout levels—level 1 if you're new to strength training, which focuses on bodyweight moves and dumbbells, or level 2, a barbell-based workout for more experienced users. Both include full-body moves that build muscle in less time.

Regardless of your level, there are workouts three times a week. Every exercise included in each workout, the combination of moves, and even the order in which you do them is intentional. Each workout is designed with muscle building in mind. The result? You get stronger and you're able to build more muscle tissue, improving your metabolism.

You'll find the workouts in the daily Core 4 challenges, but here's an example of one so you know what to expect. This level 1 workout should take thirty minutes or less to complete. Like all the workouts, it includes upper- and lower-body compound movements (plus core work!):

GOBLET SQUATS—*4 sets of 10 reps*

Stand with your feet slightly wider than hip width and hold a dumbbell or kettlebell in front of your chest. Inhale and engage your core as you hinge from your hips and bend your knees to lower your butt toward the floor, keeping your feet in a comfortable squat stance with your thighs a little lower than parallel. Exhale as you return to the starting position.

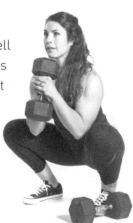

ALTERNATING LUNGES—*3 sets of 8 reps with each leg*

Stand with your feet under your hips, holding dumbbells in both hands. Step forward and bend your right knee to make a 90-degree angle with your right leg as you lower your left knee toward the floor. Drive through your front foot. Step forward with your left leg to bring your feet together. Repeat the movements on the opposite leg.

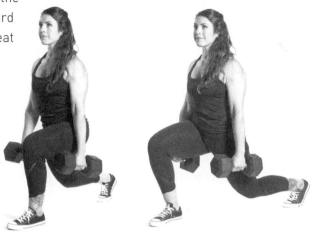

Pro Tips

» Make your step short enough that you can return to standing without swinging your torso.

» *To make it harder,* make them walking lunges, or hold the dumbbells over your head while you lunge.

PUSH-UPS—*3 sets of 8 reps*

Lie facedown on the floor and place your hands on the floor next to your body at about chest level, with your elbows close to your sides. Your body should look like an arrow if you could view it from above, not the letter T. Push your body up so that you're on your hands and toes, keeping your body in a straight line. Don't stick your butt up into the air or drop your butt too low. Bend your elbows to lower your chest toward the floor, and then push back up. As you push up, take a breath and keep your butt and core tight.

Pro Tip

» *To make it harder,* add weight on your back, or try clapping push-ups.

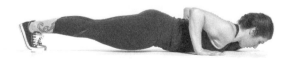

WAITER WALKS—*3 sets of 50 feet with each arm*

Stand with your feet under your hips and hold light- to moderate-weight dumbbells in each hand. Press your right dumbbell up toward the ceiling, actively pushing through your shoulder and keeping your right arm close to your head. Then walk with the dumbbell overhead. Pull your ribs down instead of flaring them out. Repeat the movements with your left arm.

SEATED SIDE TWISTS—*3 sets of 8 reps on each side*

Sit on the floor with your knees bent, your feet flat on the floor, and a dumbbell held in both hands at chest height. Lean back, bringing your feet off the floor, and slowly twist your body to the right as you move the dumbbell toward your right hip. Keep your sit bones on the floor. Then rotate your body slowly to the left, moving the dumbbell toward your left hip. Keep the weight close to your body as you rotate from side to side.

SUPER(WO)MANS OR BIRD DOGS—*3 sets of 12 reps*

Lie facedown on the floor and extend your arms out in front of you. Inhale and then exhale as you engage your core and lift your arms and legs a few inches off the floor. Activate your back and butt muscles, moving slowly until you reach a comfortable maximum height. Hold for 1 to 3 seconds, then return to the starting position.

Pro Tips

» *To make it harder*, increase the reps.

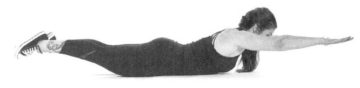

» *To make it easier*, decrease the reps, or don't lift as far off the floor. You can also substitute with bird dogs: position yourself on all fours on the floor and extend one arm out in front of you while also extending the opposite leg out behind you, keeping your weight centered; then switch the arm and leg.

MUSCLE'S MANY BENEFITS

For women, strength training has incredible benefits. It improves sleep, reduces depression, boosts mood and self-esteem, and improves bone density. It may even delay the chromosomal damage that occurs as we get older by protecting our body's telomeres, the ends of our DNA. It also helps us maintain balance and coordination and keeps our metabolism running strong.

Skeletal muscle is an endocrine tissue, which means it releases compounds that influence other tissues in the body. As you exercise, muscle cells release chemicals called myokine messengers. Some of these have a whole-body effect, upregulating fat metabolism. Said simply, when you activate more muscle by lifting weights, you increase your ability to burn fat and build muscle.

LET'S TALK CARDIO

Cardio is typically an exercise that gets your heart and breathing rates up. That could be walking, jogging, biking, swimming, Zumba—you name it. Some cardio is good for you. No doubt about it. But—and this is a big but—the kind of cardio you do matters.

You have two general types of muscle fibers: slow-twitch and fast-twitch. (Fast-twitch are actually further divided into other categories, but we'll keep it simple here.) Something like walking, which you can do for hours, primarily uses slow-twitch muscle fibers. These fibers are more fatigue resistant, allowing you to stay in motion for long periods of time—walking, sitting, reading, sleeping, whatever. The longer you can do something, the fewer fast-twitch fibers you tend to use.

Fast-twitch fibers, on the other hand, generate more power and fatigue more quickly. Your fast-twitch fibers kick in when you lift a heavy weight, sprint, or really push yourself hard physically. Think about it. You can't do these exercises for very long before you get tired and need to rest.

Bulky, Schmulky!

The one thing I hear most from women about lifting weights is that they think they'll end up big and bulky. Let's end this one for good. The way you lift causes changes in muscle fibers at the cellular level. There are two different types of muscle growth, or hypertrophy, that happen based on the lifting you do.

The first type of muscle growth is sarcoplasmic, in which more fluid is added to the muscle cell itself. The cell expands without getting proportionally stronger. This kind of weight training usually involves tons of reps and sets at lower weights to expand the fluid of the muscle fiber, producing bulk. Nobody ever accidentally ended up looking like a bodybuilder. That takes very specific training, tightly controlled nutrition, and a ton of dedication. The type of workouts in the Core 4 program are not designed for bulking.

The other type of hypertrophy is myofibrillar, in which the number of contractile proteins in the muscle is increased by doing fewer reps of more challenging weights. This may increase the size of the muscle tissue a little bit, but it primarily makes you stronger.

The type of strength training in the Core 4, with fewer reps and heavier weights, means that while you might see a slight gain in size—say, biceps definition where you didn't have it before—you're not going to look like the Hulk. Plus, it's okay to take up more space!

When you work out, you'll want to involve as much muscle as possible, because the more muscle you use, the more benefit you get. That means strength training and staying active throughout the day. And there is evidence that if you don't use those fast-twitch fibers, they may become slow-twitch over time (more on that shortly). That makes it harder to maintain your strength and move your body quickly—like if you need to catch yourself from falling.

In fact, dynapenia, or loss of power, is becoming more common and not just among the elderly. Plus, the loss of muscle tissue, called sarcopenia, has a negative impact on health, function, and longevity. In short, losing muscle is not good for your health, regardless of your age.

So when you do steady-state cardio, like when you run on a treadmill or use an elliptical machine for an hour, yes, you're burning calories. You're working your heart and cardiovascular system, but you're not using the full potential of your muscles. When you combine undereating with long cardio sessions, you may lose weight, but some of that weight is likely muscle tissue. I know this may contradict everything you believe, like, "I'm on a quest to lose weight, so I'm going to do only cardio." But if your body has to break down its own muscle to make energy, you're going to be worse off than when you started.

In general, you can lose weight in three ways:

1. By *losing water,* through dehydration or carb manipulation. The adult female body is about 55 percent water. If you lose fluids, you can lose "scale weight." But that's obviously not a sustainable long-term weight-loss strategy. Plus, the body is always working to reestablish homeostasis, including water balance. Slashing carbohydrate intake may also lead to weight loss—at first. Your body needs 3 to 4 grams of water to process each gram of carbs you eat. This explains why after a carb-heavy day of typical refined-grain pizza/pasta/bread-type meals you wake up feeling bloated—and the scale goes up. But you didn't gain fat from this overnight, and the water gain is temporary.

2. By *tapping into fat,* which happens over a longer timeframe—and is what you'll achieve in the Core 4 program.

3. By *losing muscle,* which has negative consequences for your metabolism and overall health.

The first method, losing water, is only temporary. Once you return to a normal hydration status or replenish your glycogen stores, any "losses" disappear. Losing muscle may result in a lower number on the scale, but the less muscle you have, the more your metabolism sinks. For the most sustainable health gain and body recomposition, it's important to build muscle over time using the nutrition, movement, and recovery strategies in this book.

There's another aspect to consider. Long sessions of steady-state cardio have their benefits. They help you de-stress and can lift your mood (thanks, endorphins!). But you know how the old saying goes: too much of anything isn't good for your body. Overdoing exercise—like when you do hours of cardio day after day—is stressful on the body. This leads to chronic oxidative stress, which can cause damage to DNA and cell death. It also lowers the body's antioxidant stores because it produces more free radicals. Longer, more intense, and more frequent workouts make it harder for the body to cope. Oxidative stress of this nature causes chronic inflammation, which we've seen is linked to serious illness and disease.

As I hope you'll discover for yourself, a lot of cardio without weight training isn't the answer. But if you still want to do cardio, get smart about it. Instead of slogging through sessions on the treadmill, do interval training (which we'll talk about next) or get your cardio through a challenging session of weight lifting (yes, you can do both at once!). Or, at the very least, offset your cardio sessions with weights.

A Better Way to Do Cardio: Interval Training

During the Core 4 program you'll have the option to add interval workouts to your off days each week, and if you want to do cardio along with the program, I recommend interval training.

Interval training means that instead of exercising at a slow, steady pace, you push yourself hard for a short period of time, then follow that up with a recovery period. And repeat. Those intervals can vary, but a one-to-one ratio—for example, one minute of working hard followed by one minute of recovery—is common.

When you interval train, you usually move faster and therefore use fast-twitch muscle fibers. You get the benefits of cardio without the long workout duration and higher stress. And interval training should be short and sweet, because if you do it right, you get tired!

For example, Tabata is a type of interval training developed by Japanese researcher Dr. Izumi Tabata. You do eight rounds of alternating twenty-second exercise and ten-second rest intervals. That means you go all out for twenty seconds, recover for ten seconds, and then do it again. It's incredibly hard, even though you're working for only four minutes total!

My point? You don't need an hour of interval training to get the benefits. Try a short Tabata workout. Warm up on an exercise bicycle, treadmill, or elliptical trainer for five minutes. Do four minutes of Tabata intervals—twenty seconds on, ten seconds off—and then cool down for four minutes. That's it.

Or warm up for five minutes and then do a minute of hard effort followed by a minute of recovery. Do five to ten intervals of this, then cool down.

With either interval workout, start off gradually, doing it once or twice a week.

It's worth noting that if you're experiencing adrenal, thyroid, or autoimmune issues or you're generally pretty stressed, interval training and long sessions of cardio may make those conditions worse. Opt for a few short sessions of weight training each week combined with walking or another very low-intensity movement, like walking or gentle yoga, instead, and listen to your body.

THE NEAT PHENOMENON: MOVING YOUR BODY MORE

Strength training is one aspect of this pillar, but it represents only a fraction of your day—about thirty to forty-five minutes a few times a week. How you spend the rest of your time matters. That's where NEAT, or non-exercise activity thermogenesis, comes in. This fancy term simply means that by moving your body more throughout the day—by adding non-exercise movement—you use more energy.

Examples include getting up and moving around more often during the day, sitting less frequently, doing light housework and chores, walking instead of driving, and even fidgeting. These things may not feel like exercise, but they still help you move more.

Again, your environment typically works against you. Unless you have a physically demanding job where you're on your feet all day, you may spend most of your day sitting. Recent research has found that even if you work out on a regular basis, it's probably not enough to offset the health consequences of sitting all day, every day—an average of nine to eleven hours. That's a lot of inactivity.

Get creative and see where you can sneak some non-exercise movement into your routine. Take one of my clients, Heather, who works in downtown Chicago. She commutes to work from the suburbs, taking a train and then a bus to her office. She lifts weights a few times a week, but she realized she could add more activity to her workdays by skipping the bus. Now she gets off the train and walks fifteen minutes to and from her office instead of waiting for the bus. "I'm getting an extra thirty minutes of walking a day, and I feel better," says Heather, forty-two. "Before, when I got out of work, I was stressed and tired, and now I feel good by the time I get on the train."

So take a look at your day and find ways to add more movement. Try some of the following:

Park farther from your destination (as long as it's safe).

Enlist a friend, workmate, or neighbor to take walks with you before work or during your lunch hour. You're more likely to stick with it if you have a buddy.

Set a timer at work for every thirty to sixty minutes. When it goes off, get up and stretch or move around for a few minutes.

Get your stuff done! Chores like laundry, cooking, walking the dog, cleaning, and other light housework all count as movement.

Binge-watching Netflix? Use the time to stretch or do mobility work. Even that is better than being totally inactive.

Work smarter. Try a standing desk at your office, suggest walking meetings, and stroll to someone's office instead of emailing.

THE MENTAL ASPECTS OF STRENGTH

Strength training doesn't merely have physical benefits. The real magic is what it does for your mind. Outer strength begets inner strength, and vice versa.

Now that workouts like CrossFit and American Ninja Warrior are gaining popularity, the pendulum seems to be swinging in the opposite direction, but chances are that the narrative you heard growing up was that it wasn't cool for girls or women to be strong. Even today, I see young girls climbing monkey bars, but by the time they've

started high school, that sense of physical strength, confidence, and freedom has been lost.

It's normal—natural, even—to doubt your own strength. Even in my early thirties I remember thinking, *I'm never going to be strong enough to climb a rope or do a pull-up.* I was wrong—I was eventually able to do both. But when you doubt your physical capacity, it tends to spill over into your self-confidence as well.

As you become physically stronger, your mental and emotional strength grows too. It's like a loop. There's something so empowering about facing a challenge that may scare you a little bit. Perhaps you set out to lift a weight that you're not sure you can handle. When you do it, you realize, *Hey, I did it! I didn't die!* And your brain gets a little dopamine ping. If you're getting cheered on by your workout buddies, cue serotonin too, the happiness neurotransmitter. And when you all hug it out or high-five afterward, oxytocin kicks in and strengthens your bond. Then you think, *What else can I do?*

When you prove your self-doubt wrong, that's super powerful. It's a heady, profound feeling. Here's the thing: you are innately strong. That's how you're supposed to be! You're not built to be weak. Your body and mind thrive off strength!

The physical changes of building muscle may be easy to see and measure—your body gets stronger, you start to see muscle definition you never noticed before—but you change psychologically and emotionally as well. Those changes may be harder to pin down, which is why you'll fill out a Health Tracker before and after the Core 4 program (see the "Get Ready" chapter, page 91).

As Shannon, age forty-two, says:

The [Core 4 program] was an awakening for me. I have learned so much about the "why" of my self-sabotaging behavior, which has led me to really listen to my body and actually enjoy the here and now without always worrying about the mistakes of the past and the unknowns of the future. Besides getting stronger physically, I feel emotionally and mentally stronger to set out every day and enjoy the life and body that I am blessed with . . . I finally feel free of the fear of food and the need to try to punish and control my body through rigorous and damaging exercise.

When I think of how outer strength begets inner strength, I think of the tendency to wait until we feel a certain way before we take action in our lives. You might think, *When I feel confident, I'll finally wear a swimsuit on the beach* or *When I feel motivated, I'll go to the gym.*

Instead, consider this: going to the gym and doing your workout boosts feelings of motivation. It's kind of like faking it until you make it. Break free of the loop of "I feel and then I do" and replace it with "Act how I want to feel." It might not work all the time, but you'd be surprised at how much more you can accomplish with that shift. As you strengthen your body, you build capacity and confidence and motivation. Instead of focusing on making yourself smaller, you grow stronger and increase your presence. And that makes you feel unstoppable.

BEYOND EXERCISE: TAKING CARE OF YOUR "MEAT SUIT"

As you've seen, strength training builds more muscle, skill, and confidence. But there's more to it than just lifting weights. Remember, your body gets stronger during recovery—not during strength training itself—so you cannot underestimate the importance of rest and recovery. It's common to start a workout program yet forget to take care of your body. The result is stiffness, soreness, or even injury.

Think about maintaining your body like you maintain your car. A little preventive care goes a long way. The human body is designed to move, and when you don't, your tissues get sticky and gummy, your muscles feel tight, and your joints ache. Your posture degrades and your back gets sore. When that happens, you're less motivated to move.

Yet overtraining isn't good either. You know about the drawbacks of too much cardio now and the benefits of interval training. During recovery, your body adapts to the training demands you're putting on it, and the type of recovery you need may depend on how hard you're working out. Someone who exercises six days a week might go for a walk or a bike ride on her day off but still consider that a recovery day. Another woman might lift weights three times a week and consider the days between her workouts her recovery days.

Help your body's recovery process along with practices that keep your tissues and joints flexible. This also keeps the fascia—the connective tissue sheath surrounding

your muscles and organs—healthy and pliable. Like its name implies, "active" recovery involves doing something physical that speeds adaptation, even if the activity is gentle or low-key.

Aim to include some **ACTIVE RECOVERY** once or twice a week. Options include the following:

MOBILITY WORK. This is about restoring proper body position, posture, and alignment, as well as joint range of motion. These are short, targeted interventions to improve joint movement. You'll do some of these during the Core 4 day-to-day program.

STRETCHING OR GENTLE YOGA. You can easily fit a few simple stretches, such as a doorway chest stretch and a neck stretch, into your day.

FOAM ROLLING. A foam roller lets you provide self-myofascial release. It's like giving yourself a deep-tissue massage for free! It helps resolve muscle tension and relieve trigger points.

LIGHT CARDIO. An activity such as walking, to get your body moving without intensity, promotes recovery.

PASSIVE RECOVERY. These are activities that don't require physical movement—everything from napping to saunas to cryotherapy. Try to work some passive recovery into your schedule once a week. Here are some passive recovery options:

NAPPING. This is possibly the simplest way to help your body recover. A short nap of twenty minutes or less can speed healing and recovery and shouldn't interfere with your sleep at night.

SAUNA. A twenty-minute sauna is basically a heat stressor that can ease chronic pain, promote cardiovascular health, and improve your body's normal detoxification processes. In our temperature-controlled modern environments we often don't get exposed to the more natural shifts that may prompt a process known

as hormesis, which is a fancy term for a low dose of a stressor producing a beneficial effect on the body. (Check with your doctor before you use a sauna or the next option, cryotherapy.)

CRYOTHERAPY. Just as a sauna exposes you to more extreme heat, cryotherapy uses cold to boost immune function, reduce pain and inflammation, and even increase metabolism. You can opt for a cold-water bath or stand-alone units that use super-cooled air to lower your body temperature for short bursts of time.

CONTRAST SHOWER OR BATH. This is a cheap and easy way to combine the benefits of hot and cold therapy. Take a quick hot shower (or bath) followed by a cold one to help reduce muscle soreness and speed recovery, decrease inflammation, and possibly even boost metabolism. The change in water temperature alters the blood flow between the skin and muscles and your internal organs. Use a ratio of three hot to one cold—three minutes in hot water followed by one minute in cold—and repeat three or four times, but build up to this amount over time.

EPSOM SALT BATH. This is a tried-and-true method of decreasing soreness and improving relaxation. Dissolve 1 to 2 cups magnesium sulfate—Epsom salt— in very warm bath water and soak for ten to fifteen minutes.

ACUPUNCTURE. This centuries-old practice is now more accepted by the mainstream and may reduce pain, speed healing, boost your immune system, and loosen tight muscles.

MASSAGE OR ACTIVE RELEASE THERAPY (ART). Both of these therapies can ease sore muscles, encourage healing, and lessen inflammation. Look for a trained professional to administer either.

You don't have to do all of these things, but try to make recovery a priority. Even lying down on the floor and propping your feet up on a wall for fifteen minutes can

help get fluid moving toward your heart, relieve lower back tension, and decrease swelling after sitting for a long period of time.

You're given only one body for life. Take care of it, and it'll take care of you.

These first two pillars address two elements of health, but what about the majority of your day, the time when you're not actually eating nourishing foods or moving your body? How can you get the most from your body then? By using it thoughtfully and intentionally, which leads us to the third of the Core 4 pillars, "Recharge Your Energy."

Recharge Your Energy

Managing your energy has never been more critical than it is today. If you're like most busy women I know, you're multitasking all day, struggling to get good sleep, and feeling frantic from morning to night. Modern life, especially our work environments, expects us to act like machines, chugging away virtually nonstop—with only a couple of short breaks—day in and day out.

We're expected to be "on" all the time and super productive, pumping out quality *and* quantity. It's not uncommon to have twenty browser tabs open, hopping from task to task without ever being able to focus and execute. It's no wonder we feel drained, overworked, resentful of our jobs, and like we get nothing accomplished despite spending longer and longer hours at work—and then we lack the energy to do the things we want in our personal lives.

Women are under immense pressure to *do* all and *be* all. You're supposed to cook Pinterest-worthy dinners, sculpt a perfectly hot body, be the best partner or mother, pursue your hobbies, say yes to every social event, and, often times, be the household CEO on top of all that. You're frickin' exhausted, and no amount of mimosas and manicures is going to solve that self-care crisis. You can't step into your power if your battery is always drained.

When it comes to rest, you may assume I mean sleep. That's part of it. A good night's sleep puts a big deposit of energy back into your savings account. But if all day you're making massive withdrawals and ending up in the proverbial red, eventually it'll catch up with you. Recharging is a day and night deal.

Stepping into your inner power requires equal parts energy management, self-care strategy (the stuff that truly matters), and boundary setting. It means taking time for your damn self because the truth is nobody else is going to do it for you. Recharging doesn't have to mean skipping town for a weeklong retreat, though that does sound nice, huh? The simple strategies in this chapter can be woven into your daily routine here and there to help you recoup some of that precious energy.

Multitasking has been shown repeatedly to result in lower productivity, so why do you keep doing it? And more important, how do you stop? How do you manage all the stresses of modern life so you can feel rejuvenated instead of like drained batteries? That's what you'll learn in this chapter. Balancing your energy comes down to a few basic principles and key habits around inputs and outputs. This pillar intimately connects with the others. Often what you perceive as a food or movement problem has its roots in how rested, recovered, or stressed you are. The Core 4 framework for recharging your energy focuses on

optimizing your sleep quality and quantity;

managing how you work;

recharging yourself often, with the right mix of activities and rest; and

finding ways for you to actively de-stress.

THE MISMATCH BETWEEN ENVIRONMENT AND BIOLOGY

There's a mismatch between our environment and our human biology. We've gone from a much slower, simpler pace of life to the unprecedented pace of today's world. We're blitzed with information all day every day. It's all go, go, go; hustle, hustle, hustle; we'll sleep when we're dead; and rest is for wimps. But as author Tony Schwartz says, "The way we're working isn't working."

In theory, we should spend about one-third of each day sleeping, but most of us get far less. We ignore our body's natural rhythms without recognizing the price we

pay for it. Sleep problems become a vicious cycle: the worse you sleep, the shittier you feel. Because you're so drained, you don't have the energy to move, eat well, or take care of yourself. Poor sleep affects the hormones implicated in appetite, such as leptin, ghrelin, and neuropeptide Y. That means when you don't sleep well, not only are you tired, distracted, and irritable but you may also end up with more cravings or an out-of-control appetite. When you feel like that, it's all but impossible to make nourishing food choices or have the gusto needed for a workout.

You've already learned about how to eat better and strengthen your body. Now you'll learn how to manage your energy, and it all starts with your body's circadian rhythm.

You're a biological being living in a techno-digital world, trying to cope with a system that disregards how your body works. If you've ever gone camping for a few days, you know your body can quickly adapt to the great outdoors. The sun comes up, and you're awake. You feel drowsy and ready for sleep when it gets dark—that's common when you leave your modern, brightly lit environment. However, if you're like most people, during the day you're surrounded by obnoxious fluorescent lights, computer screens, and stale indoor air. At night, instead of a gradual decrease in light exposure (which your ancestors had), you're still flooded with light—especially the blue wavelengths that tell the brain to stay awake and alert.

Let's get a little nerdy for a minute. Natural light contains different wavelengths, including blue light, which is part of the visible spectrum from 450 to 500 nanometers. When your eyes are exposed to blue wavelengths, this signal travels through the optic nerve to the suprachiasmatic nucleus (SCN) in the brain. The SCN helps regulate your circadian rhythm, signals that it's time to be awake and alert, and prevents the release of melatonin during the day. In the evening, when the sun goes down and blue light dips, that information is relayed to the SCN too. When there's little blue light, the pea-size pineal gland in your brain releases melatonin, signaling that it's time to sleep.

The screens of our computers, tablets, and phones as well as some artificial indoor lighting give off a lot of the blue wavelengths. So when you're lying in bed with your phone a few inches away from your face, your brain and your body get the signal to be alert. Blue light is even absorbed through your eyelids when your eyes are closed. In essence, we're living in near-perpetual daytime.

Now we have artificial light coming into our eyes almost constantly. Cell phones are probably the biggest culprit. A 2017 survey of 2000 Americans by the firm Deloitte found that 66 percent of people looked at their phone within thirty minutes of going to sleep. Fourteen percent looked at their phone immediately before bed. And according to a 2016 study of over 600 American adults, more smartphone use during the day and around bedtime was associated with poorer sleep quality and quantity. In other words, the more people used their phones, the worse they slept.

That constant light exposure—too much of it at night—interferes with your body's natural circadian rhythm and wreaks havoc on your sleep. There's also evidence that blue light exposure may prevent the natural dip in body temperature that normally accompanies sleep, making your sleep more restless. Improving your sleep quality is the first aspect of this pillar.

SLEEP: A NONNEGOTIABLE

Improving your energy starts with getting better sleep. Yet, more than one-third of Americans get less than seven hours of sleep a night. Even mild but chronic sleep deprivation—like sleeping four to six hours a night—is enough to negatively affect your ability to think clearly, stay mentally alert, and feel frickin' awesome.

If you want to build muscle, kick cravings, and improve body composition, getting better, more restful sleep is key. During a full night's rest, your body repairs itself, your brain becomes more efficient, and your hormones regulate themselves. It's when you consolidate and process memory. Sleep is both physical and psychological recovery. The crazy thing is that humans are adaptable, which means many of us learn to function at a lower energy level—propping ourselves up with caffeine and sugar. You forget how good it feels to have a full night of solid rest: like a badass who can take on the world.

But people are misinformed about sleep. First, they think they won't suffer any ill effects from sleep deprivation. Wrong! I was sleep-deprived for years, getting about five or six hours a night back when I was teaching. I wasn't up all night, but I never got the sleep my body needed. Being tired and never feeling completely rested became my new normal. Starting my day was a battle. I couldn't wake up without hitting the

snooze button half a dozen times, and every morning I was so drowsy. I was stuck indoors at work all day and then spent most of the evening on my cell phone and watching TV, letting blue light pour into my eyes.

This draggy, fuzzy way of operating is the norm for many others too. I swore I was fine even though I felt far from it. In that state of mild to moderate sleep deprivation, people perform as poorly on thinking tests as if they were drunk—so, quite badly. You just can't think clearly. In fact, a 2006 study comparing total sleep deprivation with sleep restriction concluded that the sleep-restricted group—who managed to get six hours of sleep a night—performed just as poorly on cognitive tests as the subjects who had stayed awake for forty-eight hours straight. Even more telling, the group that got six hours of sleep *thought* they were doing okay. Although you might feel "fine" with less sleep, you're likely impaired when it comes to tasks involving thinking, reasoning, problem solving, and more.

I know there will always be someone who swears, "Well, my aunt Mary got only four hours of sleep a night and lived to a hundred and two," but that's an exception to the rule. Most adults need between seven and nine hours of sleep.

It's not only how much you sleep but *when* you sleep that matters. Let's say you go to sleep after midnight but you still get eight hours. That might sound reasonable, but it's not nearly as good as going to sleep earlier. Here's why:

Throughout the night, your body moves through different stages of sleep that last on average about ninety minutes. You go from lighter sleep (stages one and two) into deeper sleep (stages three and four) and through the rapid eye movement (REM) stage of sleep, which is when you dream.

During deep sleep, your brain waves slow down and your muscles completely relax. You're pretty out of it. Your body releases hormones like growth hormone and prolactin (which is important for the immune system and metabolism) and repairs damaged tissues. This is when physical recovery really happens—when you're in deep sleep, your body is repairing itself, shoring up the immune system, and rebooting for the next day.

The first big chunk of deep sleep you get when you're dead to the world is spurred by the rise of melatonin, a hormone produced by the brain (in the pineal gland) that basically tells your body to go into sleep mode. Its primary job is to put the brakes on your body's adrenal output. (Hint: remember cortisol from the Pillar 1 chapter?)

When it comes to sleep, cortisol and melatonin oppose each other. Cortisol ramps up in the morning and tapers off in the afternoon, while melatonin starts to ramp up in the afternoon and peaks around 2:00 a.m. If most or all of your sleep occurs after that peak of melatonin, you miss your opportunity to get the highest-quality, deepest sleep.

As you continue through the night toward the morning hours, you get less deep sleep and more REM sleep, yet both are vital for optimal rest and recovery.

When you don't sleep enough, or you don't go to sleep at the same time every night, it's hard to develop a consistent routine. The answer? Go to bed at a reasonable time that syncs better with your circadian rhythm, and introduce regularity to your sleep-wake cycle.

The Keys to Better Sleep

When you're stuck in a crappy sleep cycle, it can be hard to break out, but addressing a few basic things can have a tremendous impact. In the Core 4 program, you'll spend a few days focusing specifically on your sleep. In the meantime, you can make these small changes:

START WITH BREAKFAST. Believe it or not, better sleep starts with your morning meal. In order to make melatonin, you need to produce serotonin, often called the "happiness" neurotransmitter.[1] Serotonin is very important to your brain, but most of it is made in your gut. One of the amino acids that helps produce serotonin is tryptophan, which is typically found in animal-based foods—most famously in your Thanksgiving turkey—but even walnuts contain tryptophan too. Start your day with a decent breakfast that includes 20 to 30 grams of protein, ideally from animal sources because they have all the essential amino acids. You'll get a dose of tryptophan, and the protein may ward off snacking or cravings later in the day because protein is so satiating.

Also, a larger breakfast will help you "front-load" your meals, meaning you take in more calories earlier in the day and have lighter meals at night for better digestion and sleep. If you're not a big breakfast person, try something light, like soup or eggs.

---

[1] Selective serotonin reuptake inhibitors, or SSRIs, which are used to treat depression, help keep serotonin around a little bit longer between your neurons. In general, more serotonin equals improved mood.

GET OUTSIDE. Ideally, aim for fifteen minutes of sunlight exposure in the morning. Sunlight helps regulate your circadian rhythm, keeping you alert during the day. Try to get a brief walking break outside before noon, without sunglasses if you can.

REDUCE CAFFEINE. You may not be able to imagine your morning without a cup (or two) of coffee. An enzyme in your liver—cytochrome P450 1A2—is responsible for processing caffeine. While some people are lucky fast metabolizers, three-quarters of the population are slow metabolizers. Keep in mind, too, that caffeine has a half-life of six hours. That means that six hours after drinking a cup of coffee, your body has metabolized only half of it, so if you drink it late in the day, it could affect your sleep.

A better bet? Swear off caffeine after noon. Try switching to caffeine-free herbal tea.

CREATE A BEDTIME ROUTINE. Signaling your body that you're getting ready to wind down and go to bed makes it easier to fall asleep. This doesn't mean rushing around for five minutes before you crawl into bed. Plan on taking thirty to sixty minutes before sleep to engage in your bedtime routine.

Stay off electronics for at least an hour before bed to avoid adrenaline spikes (looking at you, online trolls!) and blue light. Better yet, opt for low-key activities, like washing the dishes, laying out your clothes for the next day, taking a bath or shower, or reading. Everyone has their own mix, but your body and brain need more than a few minutes to wind down.

LIMIT LIGHT EXPOSURE. Light, especially the blue wavelengths, tells your brain to stay alert. In the evening, use screen-dimming programs like f.lux or Night Shift on your electronics. Also use salt lamps or candles, and install dimmers on other lamps—as the sun goes down, lower the lights in your house. Try swapping out fluorescent and LED light sources you use in the evening for bulbs with more yellow and red wavelengths. These colors are at the opposite end of the light spectrum and aren't as stimulating as blue light. (Think of the warm glow a fire gives off.) You can also try amber or blue-blocking glasses to reduce the blue light that reaches your eyes. The most inexpensive pairs start at around ten dollars.

TRY ESSENTIAL OILS. Some scents have powerful calming properties. Use an essential oil like lavender or cedarwood before you go to sleep. Essential oils have been used for centuries to relax and calm the body, and have been shown in studies to reduce anxiety and stress.

SET THE STAGE. Your bedroom should be dark, cool, and quiet. Room-darkening shades that keep out ambient light, a noise machine that masks traffic or outside noise, and a lower room temperature (between 65 and 68 degrees Fahrenheit) can all improve your sleep. Get in the habit of leaving your electronic devices, like your phone and tablet, in another room, with the sound turned off. If you need an alarm, get a regular analog alarm clock. You likely don't *need* a phone in your bedroom!

WORKING WITH YOUR ULTRADIAN RHYTHM

Sleep is one piece—possibly the most important piece—of managing your energy, but you can sleep pretty well and still have a daytime routine that leaves you drained. You're not a machine capable of working at 100 percent all the time.

When I talk about energy, I mean physical, mental, and emotional energy, all of which you can boost by working with your body's natural ultradian rhythms.

An ultradian rhythm cycle typically lasts between 90 and 120 minutes, whether you're awake or asleep, and affects your ability to concentrate, learn, and focus. You've probably experienced this when working or studying. You're able to concentrate for an hour or two, and then it's so easy to get distrac— Oh look, something shiny!

As you've seen, human biology is tied to cycles and rhythms: our appetites, sleep and wake times, hormonal fluctuations, and more. Yet the conveniences of modern life allow us to override our cycles and go full linear, working harder with fewer rest periods, flooding our homes and workplaces with artificial light, and ignoring our natural drive to eat in the name of dieting. I'm not saying we must live in caves and give up all modern conveniences, but if we do things smarter, we can make our bodies happier and healthier at the same time.

You're probably already aware of your own natural energy fluctuation. You may have noticed the peaks and troughs, ups and downs during your day. You may even know when

your most productive time of day is. My friend Kate loves to write at night because she feels less inhibited late in the day, whereas I do my best work first thing in the morning.

No matter how productive you are, at some point you'll experience energy lulls. Let's say you didn't sleep well, skipped breakfast, and had a lunch full of processed carbs. Now it's 3:00 p.m. and you're exhausted. You can't focus, you're hungry, and you feel like crap. This is the midafternoon slump that nearly all of us experience.

Now let's say you had a good night's sleep, a protein-packed breakfast, followed by a productive morning of work and a balanced lunch. It's 3:00 p.m. and you hit your afternoon slump. This isn't the time to do any focused, brain-heavy work, so you might catch up on email or take a quick walk outside. You'll still have an energy lull, but because of the way you've slept and eaten, it won't be as dramatic. Honoring your body's ultradian rhythm and giving yourself a break can help you feel heaps better.

You may be expected—or expecting *yourself*—to perform at a high level straight through the entire day. But this isn't possible when it comes to mental focus and cognitive ability. Deep, "in the zone" mental focus is not limitless. We all naturally work in these 90- to 120-minute stretches and then drift off because our ability to focus is tapped out. You may scroll social media or scan the headlines because you're looking for a break, but this isn't the kind of break that revitalizes you.

Embrace the 90-30 Workflow

This is where the 90-30 workflow comes in. It's an amalgam of some of the work of Tony Schwartz, author of *The Way We're Working Isn't Working,* corporate wellness insight from my friend Jamie Scott, and parts of the Pomodoro time-management technique. And it's simple. Do 90 minutes of work followed by a 30-minute break. The idea is that you work, rest, and repeat. When I was working on this book, I'd write for 90 minutes and then take a solid 30 minutes off to go for a walk outside or do some light chores. I didn't, however, hop on my email or keep working on a different but mentally draining task. Scrolling through email and social media is not an energizing activity. Let's be honest: it's usually way more draining!

If you have little flexibility in your workday and you rarely get a break, you can still get creative when you do have the occasional moment of downtime with something called "channel switching." If you have a mentally taxing job where you're staring at a

computer screen all day, try doing some light physical activity to reboot. That might be going outside for a 15-minute break and focusing your eyes on something distant to reduce fatigue. Maybe it's taking a walk or stretching.

If you have a job that's more physically demanding, give yourself more of a mental recharge. During an eight-hour shift, going to CrossFit on your lunch break may not be your best channel switch. A better option might be sitting down and taking a break outside, using a meditation app, reading, or something else that gives your body a rest. You have to do what's right for your routine, but see where you can find some easy energy wins in your day.

You drain yourself all day long . . . and then you wonder why you're so tired. If you use your phone all day and don't plug it in to recharge, it dies. That's a very simple closed system, but we're complex biological beings. It's more nuanced with us. **Being drained saps your willpower, and that makes it harder to choose nourishing foods and get a workout done—another way the four pillars interrelate.**

You may resist this 90-30 idea, swearing you're more productive when you just push through. But it's important to experiment with this during the next thirty days of the program. I promise you'll be amazed at how much more energized you feel. Everyone I know who has tried it has said something like "Holy shit, I've gotten way more work done than I did before!" Most people are good for about three or four of these work-rest cycles a day, which equals up to six hours' worth of focused, productive output.

GIVE UP MULTITASKING

The other major change you can make to align yourself with your body's natural energy cycles may seem counterintuitive, but I want you to try it anyway. It's this simple (but probably not easy): give up multitasking.

I know, I know. You're probably used to having multiple documents and websites open on your computer at any given time. You return calls from your Bluetooth headset in the car. You jump back and forth between composing emails and working on your latest project. You may think you're getting more done with multitasking, but it's all an illusion. You'll get more accomplished by focusing on one thing at a time.

Hopping from one task to another may make you *feel* like you're getting more done, but it makes it harder for your memory and cognition to function at their best.

Energy-Boosting Breaks

There are a variety of energizing breaks you can take as part of your workflow. (And the 90-to-30 ratio is only a suggestion—even a short break of 10 or 15 minutes can help you work with your body's natural ebbs and flows and be more productive.) Give these breaks a try:

USE A GUIDED MEDITATION. Fire up a guided meditation podcast, app, or video, pop in your headphones, and bliss out. Tons of meditations can be done in a seated position, whether you're on a park bench or at your desk.

ENJOY A CUP OF HOT TEA OR BROTH. Take the time to sip and savor a hot beverage while taking a screen break.

FIND A "SIT SPOT." Choose a place, preferably outside, and sit for ten minutes. Observe what's around you without judging, and simply let your mind wander as you breathe deeply and slowly.

CONNECT. Call someone you can connect with, and take the time to catch up over the phone. (Texting doesn't count.) Or sit and chat with a friend for a few minutes. This is a simple way to boost the feel-good neurotransmitter serotonin. Hug it out—with permission—for some bonus oxytocin, the bonding and empathy hormone.

GET GRATEFUL. Sit or walk and make a mental list of things you're grateful for, no matter how small.

DO A LIGHT WORKOUT. A quick walk or a few yoga poses or stretches will get your blood flowing and ease tight muscles.

There's something called a "switching cost." It's hard during multitasking to descend into focused thinking. The result? You're less productive.

Try to open only one document at a time, or check your email just once or twice a day, then respond to all your messages. (You may also save time in doing this because you're not constantly disrupted by pings, dings, and screen notifications.

Spend Less Time on Social Media

According to a 2017 survey, the average adult spends two hours and fifteen minutes on social media every day. It's probably higher than that now. A 2015 study clocked it at less, an hour and forty minutes, on average, but that's still a huge amount of time spent—I mean wasted—on social media.

If you've ever felt like you can't give up social media but it's also a giant time suck, you're not alone. It has to do with dopamine, a powerful neurotransmitter. Dopamine has a role in the anticipation-reward loop in your brain. It explains the feel-good thrill you experience before you pull the lever on a slot machine—or when you see the little red notification on your email or hear your phone chime with a Facebook notification.

Social media designers understand—and leverage—this powerful loop. The dings, red dots, likes, hearts, and infinitely scrollable screens become nearly irresistible to your brain so you keep checking and endlessly scrolling. (For what it's worth, I'm not immune to the tug of social media. It's probably my biggest energy management struggle.)

So how can you limit the time you spend on social media? Apps like Moment and Screen Time let you track how much you use your phone, and set limits on it as well. Apps like SelfControl let you block certain websites or social sites if they become a problem. iPhones now enable you to control screen time too.

Turn off all the screen and sound notifications you can, and silence your phone and computer if possible. You may also want to keep your phone away from your desk entirely since its mere presence can be extremely tempting and distracting.

Distraction central.) Or give yourself a physical cue that it's time to focus. I put on my big noise-canceling headphones, and when I do that, I know it's work time.

MANAGE YOUR STRESS BETTER

Aligning your sleep cycle with your circadian rhythm and your workday with your ultradian rhythm are two components of managing your energy. The third is learning how to handle stress.

If you get great sleep but then feel like a hunted deer all day long, you're going to feel exhausted. Mental and emotional stress—and even too much physical stress, like overexercising—is super draining. Whether you're worrying about money, dodging energy vampires, doing a job you hate, eating too little, or not recovering enough from exercise, you might sleep like a champ but still drag through your day.

Cortisol surges, which you learned about earlier, need to be balanced by rest and recovery. The pressures of modern life to be "on" all the time and to contend with unchecked stress can have negative outcomes you might not expect, such as increased cravings, low sex drive, and chronic infections.

It's all about *defusing* stress when it happens, not crafting a stress-free life. Much like strengthening a muscle, when we experience a healthy amount of stress and recover from it, we get stronger. Too little stress can lead to a failure to thrive whereas too much stress can lead to burnout. Limiting unnecessary stressors, getting clear about what's in your control (and not), and adding stress relievers to your routine are all vital.

Positive stress—technically called eustress—is something that provides a benefit. A very simple example is lifting weights. During a strength training session, your muscles sustain microscopic tears. Your body repairs this damage and you recover from the stress. The key is that you back off and allow for recovery. That's how you get stronger.

What you experience as eustress is personal. For example, the idea of embarking on a solo trip around the world may be exciting and stressful in a good way for you, prompting you to put your finances in order, renew your passport, and get the right vaccinations. On the other hand, the idea of traveling itself—let alone around the world!—could be utterly paralyzing.

There are so many kinds of stress. As you saw from the previous example, exercise can be a source of stress, especially if you work out too intensely or too often. Food can be a stressor if you're eating those foods that irritate your gut or cause inflammation, like sugar, vegetable oils, and processed foods. Constant worry and anxiety about dieting is also a stressor, as are environmental toxins, crazy relationships, and even positive life events like getting married or buying a house.

My point? You need to balance it with recovery. One way is to turn down the sympathetic nervous system and tap into the parasympathetic nervous system

instead. When you find yourself getting lost in a loop of stress, what I call "brain drain," the cycle of negative thinking can spiral out of control fast. You start to think, *I suck, my life sucks, everything sucks . . .* You quickly get overwhelmed. And when you're overwhelmed, it's impossible to think clearly, calmly, or creatively.

Instead, turn on your parasympathetic system—just as you do before you eat. A simple way to do this is to change the way you breathe. Diaphragmatic breathing, or belly breathing, activates the vagus nerve, which travels all the way from your gut to your brain stem. (In fact, it's the longest nerve of the autonomic nervous system.) This diaphragmatic breathing technique is powerful, plus you can do it anywhere and nobody will even know.

I like to sit, soften my belly (no sucking it in!), and breathe deeply, letting my belly expand out. I picture my diaphragm—the sheet of muscle under the lungs—descending down toward my belly button like an elevator, and I bring in as much air as I can through my nose. Sometimes I hold it briefly—counting anywhere from one to four—then I slowly release the breath through my nose, imagining my diaphragm traveling back up toward my heart. Try to do at least five of these deep breaths when you feel yourself getting stressed.

Stop, Breathe, and Do

The body's stress response meant survival or death in our hunter-gatherer days. But in the modern world, you're more likely to worry about money, relationships, your health, the future, the planet, or hitting your macros—rather than fighting off a predator. These worries are amplified, and instead of being brief, they're often unrelenting. When you live under chronic stress, your body constantly releases blood sugar, then churns out insulin to deal with it. Chronic stress and inflammation are linked with diseases, including cardiovascular disease, type 2 diabetes, and cancer.

In response to stress, you can put the brakes on your sympathetic nervous system and instead engage the parasympathetic by taking what I call an SBD—stop, breathe, and do—break.

You *stop* by being present where you are, checking in with your body to feel areas of tension, and recognizing that you're not in any physical danger. Pay attention to your body's stress signals. Some people get a sick feeling in their gut. Others notice that

their breathing gets shallow, or they feel tense in their shoulders and neck. I get a tight feeling in my throat. When I notice it, I tap my fingertips together to help me get back into my body and remember that I'm *right here* instead of caught up in the maelstrom in my head. My friend Erin focuses on the sensation of her feet being rooted to the ground to get physically present.

Next, you *breathe* by engaging in diaphragmatic belly breathing, which stimulates the parasympathetic rest-and-digest system and lowers the stress response.

And finally, you *do* by engaging in something creative, using your hands, and/or doing something you enjoy. You might work in your garden, write in your journal, chop vegetables for dinner, sing, or play a musical instrument.

Stress closes off your thinking like virtual blinders, but taking an SBD break expands your mind to see more possibilities. These kinds of breaks help restore your energy and give you the room to disengage from stress. The point isn't to have zero stress forever but to limit chronic stress and defuse the stress you do experience. Work actively to reduce the stressful things in your life, including taking junk food out of your diet and replacing it with nourishing food. Declutter your home or workspace, avoid energy vampires, or start a simple daily ritual like gratitude journaling.

Often the stress we face is self-created. Sometimes it can't be helped, but a lot of the time we worry about shit that doesn't truly matter. All it takes is a shift in perspective—which might sound simple, but it's not always easy.

While we've been focusing on how you eat, how you move, and how to manage your energy, we're about to change gears again—and look inside. In the next chapter, you'll learn about the importance of your mind and how to shift your outlook for the better.

PILLAR 4

Empower Your Mind

While this is the final pillar of the Core 4 program, it's crucial to all the pillars that came before it. The fourth pillar is going to change everything.

When it comes to stepping into your power, mindset is the catalyst that can turn a tiny spark into a full-on blaze. It's impactful shit. But it's also messy, nuanced, and layered. I'm not the world's foremost expert on mindset. But I *am* someone who knows from personal experience that you can look "healthy" on the outside but still benefit from work on the inside. I've used these strategies in my own life and with my clients in conjunction with the other pillars, and the strides people make are incredible. This process of exploring mindset sometimes feels like "sitting in the soup." It can be uncomfortable at times. It's also where the magic happens if you're willing to show up and do the work. But that work is never truly done—and that's not only normal, it's okay. Your perspective shifts as you change, grow, learn, and evolve. But once you become aware of your thought processes, start to challenge your self-limiting beliefs, and develop some key skills, you'll experience the transformative potential of your mind.

As you dig through this chapter and begin this work, you may find yourself questioning and evaluating your choices, where you put your energy, and what you focus

on. That's all a normal reaction. Inevitably, women ask me, "Should I keep doing XYZ?" Asking for permission usually means you're feeling disempowered. So here's a way to flip that question to put the power back in your own hands: *Is this worth what it's costing me?* Everything has a cost, whether it's your time or your energy, and whether that cost is physical, mental, emotional, or spiritual. Only you can truly know whether the trade-off is worth it. Focus on your gut reaction to that question. The gut doesn't lie, sister. That's your intuition, your inner knowing, and it's powerful AF. She's been waiting to welcome you back.

How you view the world around you, and how you choose to react to your life circumstances, is mindset in a nutshell. Do you often worry about things outside your control? Do you stay grounded when life throws things your way? Your mindset has a big impact on whether or not you'll stick with healthy eating, make movement something you look forward to, and set aside time to recharge your batteries. So let's get real about empowering your mind.

The framework for this pillar is all about

taking action on your self-limiting beliefs;

identifying your values;

building resilience;

looking for meaning outside yourself; and

determining what habits you want to change as part of the Core 4 program.

Changing your perspective isn't always easy to do—and it's not your fault if you haven't worked on any of this yet! Take the blame off yourself, and dive in with an open mind. That said, sometimes professional help is required. There's no shame in seeking therapy or coaching to work through challenging feelings.

REFRAMING YOUR BELIEFS

Your beliefs are at the core of what makes you *you,* but you probably don't spend much time thinking about them. And even if you want to, you're likely too busy with the everyday hustle of life to do so. To identify those beliefs—and whether they're holding you back—means having the willingness to examine them.

That's where the other three pillars support this fourth one. It starts with the physical. Sometimes it's more tangible to cook a meal, take care of your body, or get in a good workout before you can start to address your beliefs and values.

You may be familiar with Maslow's hierarchy of needs, where things like safety, food, and shelter have to be met before you can address "higher" needs like self-actualization. I see things in a slightly different way.

When you look at this graphic of concentric circles, imagine you're continually moving back and forth between these different aspects of your life. Addressing your body's basic physical needs first can create the foundation that lets you tunnel deeper into the core of what may be holding you back from living the life you want.

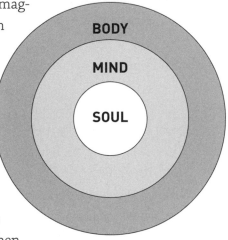

You wouldn't expect a plant to grow and thrive without sufficient sunlight, soil, and water. Well, you often must feed and water yourself to have the energy to dive deeper. It's nearly impossible to will yourself to be better or to change, especially when you don't feel good.

You learned in the previous chapter about the importance of taking SBD—stop, breathe, and do—breaks to manage stress and boost your energy during the day. You can do something similar to tune in to your inner voice.

Think about that inner voice—we all have one. What does it say? You may already have a sense of it. Maybe you know you tend to criticize yourself, or you tend to avoid taking risks, or you tend to give up on projects before you finish them. These are all self-limiting beliefs—but just because you think them doesn't make them true. Nor does it mean that they can't be changed. You get to choose which thoughts, if any, to act on and which to observe and let pass by.

The first step is to become aware of *what* that inner voice is telling you. Put the brakes on, interrupt the system, and give yourself some time to get quiet and tune in. It's like tuning a radio dial until you hear the signal clearly through the static.

Take a minute to breathe and listen. Ask questions. Get curious. When you catch yourself thinking something about yourself, ask, *Why do I believe this? Where does this*

belief come from? Is this really true? Am I playing out something from the past? Taking some time to question the thought and performing this inquiry may reveal that it is in fact untrue or unhelpful.

Your inner voice is constantly telling you things, some of which isn't true or helpful. No one can completely stop the chatter. Yet a lot of people operate under the idea of "I had this thought, so it must be true, and I must act on it." We elevate thoughts to the level of absolute truth. But we can have thoughts without accepting them as truth—or acting on them.

The Core 4 program forced Jaclyn, age thirty-one, to confront her inner voice and the damage it was causing her:

> I didn't know that it would be mindset. It caught me off guard. But it truly is where most of my problems were. I shamed myself in the mirror, in my head, about food choices, I cried about having to go to work and making bad choices (I work in a restaurant). About people seeing me that I had not seen in some time because I had gained the weight back. Food and choices and the negative voice in my head had consumed me in almost every aspect of my life. I hardly wanted to be intimate with my husband because I thought, *How could he really want this?* It took all my effort to overcome the voice.

Jaclyn developed awareness of her inner voice. The same technique works for emotional responses. If you feel defensive or offended or jealous about something, put on the brakes and question why. *Why am I so offended?* Or *What's going on in me that I feel threatened or upset about this?* It takes practice—you're probably used to simply reacting. I know I was. I was always so quick to fly off the handle when things didn't go my way, or I'd come completely undone and shame-spiral out of control if someone said something unkind to me. I couldn't even pause to see the situation as an observer, to consider the interaction before having to get a word in edgewise or defend myself. These days, things are quite different. Do I still get hurt and upset? Sure. I'm human. But more often, I'm able to pause and have awareness that hurtful words slung my way aren't actually about me in the first place and the nagging, unkind voice in my head isn't *my* voice, just *a* voice.

Yes, feel the feeling—don't bottle it up—but if it keeps bothering you, take time to tune in to those emotions. This lets you question them and recognize that there may be something deeper going on that's causing your discomfort. If you're a little scared

but also excited, that's a good thing. But if you're terrified without the excitement and suddenly feel sick to your stomach, it's worth pausing before jumping into this work. Intuition could be telling you something.

Look at this process like changing your glasses. You've been wearing an outdated prescription, and now you're going to look through new lenses. Certain things you can't change—very easily or at all. Seeing things clearly allows you to accept your reality and work to change things in the present from a place of self-respect and self-compassion. When I finally accepted and saw myself clearly, I realized I had spent decades wanting the skinny legs I saw in magazines. It wasn't worth what it had been costing me in terms of mental, emotional, and physical energy, so I let that shit go. Gratitude, that is, really practicing that feeling and honing it, is one of your best tools to shape your outlook. Can you be grateful for your body? Can you see and appreciate your strengths? Work with those. How helpful is it to focus so hard on your perceived flaws? Where can you show yourself more kindness and respect?

One of my favorite sayings is "You've survived 100 percent of your worst days." You can't change what's happened to you in the past. Wanting to get back to where you were before often digs up feelings of guilt and shame. On the other hand, focusing too hard on the future can mean you feel anxious about "not being there yet." In either case, you can't be present. It's not wrong to want to change things—your body, habits, thought patterns—but the more you focus on what was ("I want to get my body back") or what should be ("I should have lost the weight by now"), the harder it becomes to stay grateful for *what is* right now and make the choices that will move you forward. Staying engaged in the process and doing the work are what bring results. You might be thinking, *I should have started this years ago. I'm so far behind where I should be.* Stop should-ing all over yourself. You're in the perfect spot right now because *you're ready.* All you truly have is right now, so make the most of it!

You *can* change your attitude and your outlook. You can acknowledge and accept what's happened without letting it drive how you see the world forevermore. You can rewrite your story, whether it's "I've done every diet and they've never worked" or "I can't go for that promotion because I've never had that kind of responsibility before."

Bottom line: You are not your thoughts. When you learn to reframe your beliefs, to be curious about and question them, you can let go of self-limiting thoughts. That's one of the steps to unleashing your inner badass.

IDENTIFYING YOUR VALUES

Identifying thoughts that are holding you back is part of this pillar. Another aspect is identifying your personal priorities by doing a values assessment. A lot of us make choices based on something that happened in the past. At the same time, we worry

---

Values Inventory Worksheet

The following is a list of values. Start by circling twenty terms that best represent what really matters to you right now. If there are any you feel are missing, write them below the list. Don't worry about what the definition or standard meaning of a value is. It's what you interpret it to mean that matters more.

Values

Achievement	Family	Knowledge	Routine
Adventure	Financial security	Living simply	Self-respect
Balance	Freedom	Love	Self-worth
Beauty or aesthetics	Friendship	Loyalty	Social status
Comfort	Fun	Nature	Spirituality
Community	Giving to society	Passion	Success
Competition	Health	Persistence	Teamwork
Confidence	Honesty	Personal growth	Trust
Control	Humility	Power	Variety or change
Creativity	Influence	Recognition	Wealth
Education	Integrity	Relationships	Wisdom
Emotion	Intuition	Risk-taking	Other
Expertise	Job satisfaction		

After you've identified your top twenty values, narrow down your list to the five or ten that are the most important to you right now. Go a step further and group the circled values into two categories: internal, like creativity, and external, like recognition. List them on the opposite page.

too much about the future. That overthinking is paralyzing. It's one of the reasons you may *want* to change but can't manage to start. When you know what your values are, you can make decisions that align with them.

Internal Values

_____

_____

_____

External Values

_____

_____

_____

Now you've identified what really matters to you—your core values. Are you more motivated by internal or external values, or is it a mix of the two? External values are based on outside factors, like achievement or monetary success. Internal values are inherent qualities, like self-worth, love, and loyalty.

In our attainment-driven society, we tend to be motivated by status, achievement, and money. (Gee thanks, dopamine.) That stuff may be important, but external values like these are dependent on things that can be easily taken away. Internal values are innate and more often within your control.

Once you've identified your top values, rate on a scale of one to ten (one is low, ten is high) how fulfilled or satisfied you are by each of your original twenty values right now. Write the number next to each value you circled in the list. Now you have a clear picture of what's important to you, at least at this point in time, and whether you're putting time and energy into your values.

Let's say creativity is one of your top values but you're not doing anything creative at home or at work. You probably feel a disconnect there. Maybe you can't be super creative at your job, but you could start writing poetry again or take an art class. When you honor your values and put time into them, you align your life with the things that matter, and that has a profound impact.

THE BALANCE BETWEEN OUTER AND INNER FOCUS

Changing your lifestyle requires some inward focus, which is what drives and motivates you. But too much of it isn't always a good thing. Connecting to a higher purpose—something outside yourself—really matters too. You probably picked up this book because you want to work on self-improvement and ultimately embrace yourself for who you are, but there has to be equilibrium between inwardly focusing on yourself and outwardly focusing on others.

A constant inward focus can amplify any flaws or feelings of failure you have . . . and make you forget that there's a whole world outside you! If you're always focused on others, however, you may tend to get overextended and give too much of yourself. Ignoring your own health and well-being means you can't care for others to the best of your ability. We have these two dynamics opposing each other, and most people I work with struggle to find balance—they're either too focused on themselves, which leads to feelings of isolation and lack of fulfillment, or too focused on others, leaving them drained and frazzled.

The key is to establish harmony. Instead of blindly giving yourself away, focus on giving to others when it's in alignment with your values. Nobody will protect your energy for you, and sometimes that means making tough choices. Your values can help you identify your purpose, which can be something you feel drawn to—something you love to do and something that simply makes you feel good. Maybe it's volunteering or community activism. It could be picking up an old hobby for the sheer joy of it, taking the time to help a neighbor or friend in need, or simply finding time for quality connections with your loved ones.

As your values shift over the years, your purpose may too. Let's say you started volunteering at an animal shelter years ago. You started out because you love cats and want to help them. Now, six years later, you're burned out. Or you simply don't feel passionate about it anymore. Whatever the reason, it doesn't make sense for you to continue to volunteer anymore. Just because you made that commitment doesn't mean you have to continue to do it. If it doesn't align with your purpose, it's okay to let it go. Working through this process can help you choose the things that will make you happier overall.

People often try to find ways to make themselves happy from the inside, but it's critical to connect with others. As humans, we are social, and doing things for the

members of our communities gives us something that's hard to get from doing things solely for ourselves, namely serotonin and oxytocin. We try desperately in this modern world to manufacture a sense of meaning, but it's hard to get it from ourselves. Consider looking outward and connecting with others who share common values. As the saying goes, "Me to we."

If you're still not sure about your purpose, ask yourself what you love doing—what you would do even if you didn't get paid for it. What do you enjoy about it? Who do you like to do it with? How could you do more of it? How could you fit it into your schedule—if not every day, every week or month? Service to others and finding purpose can help you feel more fulfilled, boost your mood, and improve your outlook. In short? Doing good feels damn good.

Think about what's important to you and what change you can effect in the world around you. It's impossible to say yes to everything. Instead, spend your energy and time in specific ways that fit with your values and your purpose. Saying no and setting boundaries can be hard at first, but it's absolutely essential to find that harmony between caring for yourself and caring for others.

YOUR PERSONAL PILLAR PLAN: PREPARING FOR ACTION

Earlier you identified your values. Now you're going to drill down a little deeper and get more focused about habits you want to change during the Core 4 program. The Personal Pillar Plan will help you clarify where you're at right now with your pillars and decide what changes you want to make and why. Setting intentions that align with your *why* is one of the aspects of lifestyle change that's often missed, and it has a huge influence on your success in the longer term.

This kind of self-analysis is important because it's easy to exaggerate how good or bad something is if you try to guess. You might think, *Well, my nutrition sucks,* but when you take a closer look, you may see that you're actually eating pretty healthfully during the day even though you struggle with junk food at night. (This is pretty common!) Or maybe you think your energy is good because you get good sleep, but then you realize you could tweak the kind of breaks you take at work.

When it comes to overall health and wellness, people think diet and exercise are the only things that matter. Completing your Personal Pillar Plan encourages you to

change your point of view. Energy and mindset are equally as important. When you look at all four pillar areas, choose one or two things from each pillar to work on. Maybe it's putting your phone on the charger in the living room when you eat. Or

Personal Pillar Plan

In this activity, you'll gain clarity about which of the Core 4 pillars you feel is the most out of balance. From there, you'll brainstorm simple actions you want to commit to during the program. Later in the program, you'll revisit and revise. Choosing your actions strengthens autonomy and self-motivation, so don't pick what you think someone else wants you to do; pick what feels good, what's aligned for you, and what you're willing to change.

Part 1: The Core 4 Pillars

Decide whether each pillar is a 1 (needs a lot of work), 2 (needs a moderate amount of work), or 3 (needs little to no work). Then, create a bar graph for the height of each pillar.

Personal Pillar Plan graph

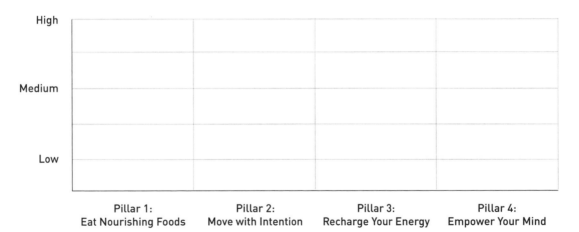

Part 2: The Pillar Actions

If you ranked a pillar a 1, come up with two simple actions you will commit to practicing each day related to that pillar. If you ranked a pillar a 2, come up with one action. And if you

adding an extra serving of veggies to your breakfast plate . . . or just *eating* breakfast. It could be doing ten side bends every time you take a bathroom break or listening to an uplifting or educational podcast while you wash the dishes.

---

ranked a pillar a 3, you may not need any new actions for now. The point is to plan to do a few positive, powerful, but simple actions each day without overwhelming yourself. Some of the lines may be left blank. Keep the focus on what you *want to do*.

Example

PILLAR 2: Move with Intention

RANK: 1 / ②/ 3

ACTION: Take a ten-minute walk in the morning before I have my coffee.

PILLAR 1: Eat Nourishing Foods

RANK: 1 / 2 / 3

ACTION: _____

ACTION: _____

PILLAR 2: Move with Intention

RANK: 1 / 2 / 3

ACTION: _____

ACTION: _____

PILLAR 3: Recharge Your Energy

RANK: 1 / 2 / 3

ACTION: _____

ACTION: _____

PILLAR 4: Empower Your Mind

RANK: 1 / 2 / 3

ACTION: _____

ACTION: _____

At the midpoint as well as at the end of the program, you'll revisit the Personal Pillar Plan and think about what has happened throughout the month. This gives you the big picture of what's changed and where there's room for improvement.

Reassessing is another opportunity to say, "Okay, here's where I am now. Where do I want to be going forward?" It's not there for you to beat yourself up if you haven't made enough progress. Lifestyle change is often anything but linear. It usually takes time and tweaks and iteration and detours to arrive where you want to be. That's why they call it a journey.

Progress is often only visible when looking back at all the small adjustments you've made and how they add up. It's not always from big, sweeping changes. When I was training for my first triathlon years ago, I had to learn to swim in open water instead of in the safety of the YMCA pool. I was terrified and out of shape. That first swim in San Diego Bay was so far outside my comfort zone that I almost didn't show up. I left the shore and quickly became very tired, stopping to tread water. The swim coach came up alongside me and said, "Even if you have to dog-paddle, you'll still move forward." That lesson has stuck with me for all these years. Baby steps are okay because you keep moving, even if it's slow going!

MAKING THE CORE 4 PROGRAM WORK FOR YOU

There's another aspect of the Core 4 program to consider before you launch into it: whether moderation or an all-or-nothing approach is a better fit for you. The all-or-nothing approach is what's found in most diets (don't eat this for twenty-one days or a month or . . . *ever*), and it's tricky. It means you can't listen to your body or your instincts about what really works for you. It means some outside source is the dictator of what's good for you, or not, and it's one of the biggest reasons women feel disempowered and confused when it comes to food and fitness.

On the other hand, some people do really well when they avoid foods or situations that are triggers, so a moderate approach might not work for everyone. Learning to listen to your body and tap into your innate inner wisdom often takes a combination approach that's unique to you. If your intuition is out of practice, that's okay. Like a muscle, it can be strengthened over time when you commit to using it.

The Core 4 program is designed to be personalized, which is what makes it successful. So ask yourself what strategy will work for you going forward. Let's say you know you're overdoing it on sugary foods and you want to break yourself of the habit of reaching for chocolate or candy when you're bored or tired. Should you make a bright-line rule and avoid all sugar forever? Or can you adopt a more moderate approach that gives you more wiggle room? That's something only you can answer. Are you more of a moderator or an abstainer? We tend to think we're all one way or all another, but humans are very complex. I have clients who are all-or-nothing people when it comes to fitness and more moderate when it comes to food.

And it can get granular. For example, I moderate chocolate just fine—I can have a couple of squares of dark chocolate without wanting to eat the whole bar—but I feel better when I abstain from alcohol entirely because alcohol lowers inhibitions, and then I make choices that aren't in line with my values. (Oh, and the headaches. Ugh.) My mental framework with alcohol is "I choose not to drink," not "I can't drink." See how those are different?

So how do you figure out what will work for you? Just as you did with your thoughts, get curious. Slow down. Listen. Check in with yourself. Ask yourself whether or not something is working. It takes self-reflection and analysis to figure out what's working and what's not, and the willingness to try something different. And that may change over time. There are aspects of personality that are pretty hardwired, but what works for you now might not work for you in a year. Allow yourself the flexibility to try something for a while, see if it's working, and if it's not, change direction. That requires you to focus on what's happening now. Don't focus so much on the future that you can't get clear about what's helping you in the present.

Keep in mind that the Core 4 program is a kick-start for the rest of your journey and a framework to encourage you to experiment, be curious, make mistakes, and then shift direction as needed. It gets pretty messy when your self-worth—how good you feel you are as a person—gets wrapped up in your need to eat or work out perfectly. As I mentioned before, this isn't a test to see how good of a rule follower you are. It's about having a life that is well lived.

The most resilient people have the ability to adjust, to learn, and to try new things. Someone yells, "Plot twist!" and they shift. Discipline alone doesn't produce results.

Neither does being too flexible. You have to balance the two. You can't be overly rigid, but if you're too flexible and never have any discipline, you won't be able to follow through with any kind of behavior change. The key is owning your choices and taking responsibility for what may come as a result.

As your resilience—that badassness—grows, you understand that perfection isn't necessary to make real, lasting progress; you realize that making a less-than-optimal choice doesn't mean you've screwed it all up, that you *can* get started again with the next meal or workout; and you're able to find health in the gray areas of everyday life instead of leaning on the strict rules of a diet plan to "keep you in line," only to fail when the 30 days are over and real life comes crashing down on you.

That's the outlook I hope you will aspire to, one that is confident yet realistic. It's normal to want to run away from things that make you uncomfortable. But true growth happens when you come up against something uncomfortable and keep walking toward it.

In the next chapter, you'll learn how to prepare for the Core 4 program. It will give you new frameworks for looking at old problems and will help put power back into your hands. So let's get started!

THE CORE 4 PROGRAM

Get Ready

Now that you've set a foundation and understand more about how the Core 4 will play a crucial role in your life, **it's time to take action**. This is the segue into the Core 4 program, which gives you a specific action to do every day for 30 days, along with meal plans and workouts to accomplish so you can start achieving the goals you set out for yourself in the previous chapter. Consuming information helps, as does having a framework, but ultimately you have to take action to succeed. And these next 30 days will be *packed* with action.

ACTION MATTERS: DOING VERSUS THINKING

It's great to get dreamy in your head about what you want, but the trick to accomplishing big goals is to *do* things instead of just thinking about them. These things may very well put you outside your comfort zone. Embrace the discomfort. Push the boundaries a little. It's how you'll grow. You'll get the most out of this program if you follow through and *take action every single day*.

I designed the Core 4 program with the idea of taking action and trying out new lifestyle tools little by little. At the end of the 30 days, you'll walk away with a toolbox

full of strategies to use whenever you're seeking to improve or change or grow. You never know what's really going to stick until you give it a whirl, which is why these 30 days are an action-packed first step on your journey.

I mentioned what you'll achieve by the end of the 30 days, and I want to highlight some of that for you here. Hopefully knowing what's waiting for you on the other side of this journey will keep you moving forward and give you the confidence to continue when things get tough.

On Day 31:

> You'll have transformed how you eat, with a focus on nutrient-dense protein, fruits and vegetables, and fats, and you'll have a framework to help you customize what you eat based on making your unique body feel great.

> You'll no longer feel blood sugar spikes and crashes throughout the day, and you'll have eliminated cravings for processed junk food.

> You'll have conquered at least fourteen challenging workouts and have a plan for continuing to build strength and flexibility.

> You'll have tools to get you to the end of your workday with energy to spare and to get the most restful sleep ever.

> You'll know how to prepare meals for the week and keep your fridge stocked with yummy, nourishing food.

> You'll have a strategy for reframing and clearing away negative thoughts when they strike.

> You'll have more focus, understand what's important to you, and know how to set actionable goals that get results.

> You'll have participated in daily health practices, from mindfulness and strength training to restful sleep and posture improvement, that will be your guiding light to lifelong health once the 30 days are over. They'll be available to you whenever you need them because your journey is ongoing.

PREPARE FOR SUCCESS

Before you start, I want you to think about the most important people in your life. I'm going to guess that you're not traveling to a remote retreat for the next 30 days—though that does sound pretty nice. If you share a home with others—family members or even a roommate—let them know that you're going to be doing something out of the norm. If you start the next 30 days expecting everyone around you to magically be on board, that may not work out very well. Having a conversation up front with the people you live with about what you're doing and why can save you from a lot of frustration later.

Look at this conversation as coming to an agreement with them instead of expressing your expectations about how they should behave. You may think people around you should be understanding and supportive, but they may not comprehend why you're making these changes. So sit down and talk it out. You might say, "I'm doing this because . . . " and "This matters to me because . . ." Explain that you'll be making some changes in the next 30 days and you'd appreciate their support. You can't guarantee how they'll react, but clear communication goes a long way.

A big reason people continue to struggle with lifestyle change is that they experience too much friction in their home environment, and over time, they give up. What you're about to do with the Core 4 might be considered unusual by the people around you, so preparing them may help.

Once you have the buy-in from those closest to you, consider what kind of equipment you may need in order to be successful with the program. Do you need a Crock-Pot to save time cooking nourishing meals? Is there other kitchen equipment you'll need—like a cutting board and a good sharp knife? I personally like a cast-iron skillet to cook with. A few simple tools are a big help. Keep reading for more specifics.

You will also need access to at least one set of dumbbells for the Core 4 workouts. If you've never exercised before or it's been a while, you can start with bodyweight exercises. Consider purchasing a couple of sets of dumbbells: one set light or medium in weight for upper-body exercises and one set medium or heavy in weight for lower-body exercises. For most women new to exercise, a set of 5- to 10-pound dumbbells and another of 15 to 20 pounds should work. If you're planning to do the level 2 program,

you'll need a barbell and some plates, and having a pull-up bar and a squat rack helps. Your local gym should have everything you need.

Think about whether you want some external accountability during the program. Some people do fine without it; some need support from others to be successful. Consider times in the past when you've taken action to change your habits. If you succeeded, did you have support or go it alone? If it's the former, ask a friend or family member to be your accountability buddy to help keep you on track.

STOCK YOUR KITCHEN

You already know that I don't believe in strict diets. That said, you *will* find some suggested meal plans in the next few chapters as you move through the Core 4 program, with recipes based on the nourishing foods listed in the Pillar 1 chapter. The most important reason I'm giving you these meal plans is that I want you to see what 30 days of eating nourishing foods can look like. The first step is to do some meal prep. You'll find my best tips for meal prepping on pages 95–100 so you can build a strategy that works for you. I suggest, also, that you stock up on nourishing foods before you start the program. Having enough on hand to make quick meals and snacks means you'll be ready in a pinch and gets you in the habit of eating these foods more often.

The weekly meal plans have these key features:

- Meals to prep, which I suggest dividing between one large cook-up day, preferably on the weekend, and a small cook-up day sometime midweek

- Breakfasts

- Lunches

- Dinners

When a meal plan says "eat leftovers," it means you're not cooking that fresh but rather having another serving of what you prepared a previous day. The meal plans also include other foods that don't have specific recipes, such as roasted cauliflower and chicken sausage. Feel free to get creative here.

These meal plans are based on a basic real-food template, so you may need to adjust for your own preferences or food sensitivities. Please substitute foods you can't or won't eat.

I don't want you to stress about counting grams of this and grams of that. You don't have to analyze, track, log, or journal your food intake. Rather, I want you to get in touch with your body's senses of hunger and fullness. Pay attention to how you feel after meals and use common sense. If you need to snack, eat a small portion of protein, carbs, and fat. You may need to up your portions at mealtime if you find you're constantly hungry. Start with a little more protein and go from there.

MEAL PREP

Picture this: It's 7:00 p.m. on a Monday night at the end the longest workday ever. You get through the front door and collapse into a heap on the sofa without even taking off your coat. Your eyes close and you enjoy a few quiet moments, letting the stress of the day melt away. And then your eyes fly open as you realize there's nothing in the fridge for dinner and you're exhausted. You eye your phone next to you on the couch and think, *Oh yes . . . pizza.* You open the meal delivery app, find your local greasy pizza joint, and . . . *(insert sound of screeching brakes here)* . . .

Oh hell no. It's not going down like that! Not this time.

From what you've learned so far, you know that willpower is drained throughout your day—hello, Mondays!—and stress increases food cravings. It's precisely in these moments that you're prone to making food decisions that you swore you wouldn't—and that you don't really want to make. So what's a gal to do? Enter meal prep. It's a foundational habit that can completely change your health for the better.

Let's finish that story with an alternate ending . . .

You open the meal delivery app, find your local greasy pizza joint, and then remember you've got a fridge full of gorgeous, satisfying food you prepped ahead of time. Food that's not going to leave you feeling sluggish and bloated. You set the phone down, take a few minutes to heat up your dinner instead of starting a meal

from scratch, and settle in for an episode of your latest Netflix fave. Dinner is delicious and satiating, and you stuck to your healthier eating plan.

Crisis averted.

The Basics of Meal Prep

The idea of meal preparation may conjure up images of twenty-one identical plastic food containers full of dry grilled chicken breast and bland steamed broccoli. Hardly appealing. If that's your perception of meal prep, allow me to blow your mind. It doesn't have to be like that at all. By spending a couple of hours in the kitchen each week, you'll efficiently stock your fridge with nourishing dishes that will get you through The Great Pizza Crisis of Monday Night and other such food emergencies. A good meal-prep session will help you get a start on lunches, cover dinners on crazy-busy nights, and take some of the pressure off when you're tired.

You can certainly use the recipes in this chapter as meal-prep staples for your busy week—Apple Braised Pork Shoulder (page 279) and Hearty Tuscan Kale Soup (page 264) immediately come to mind. But rather than tell you exactly what to make when, I'm going to share something far more useful: a meal-prep strategy that you can adapt no matter your food preferences, number of family members, or health goals.

Think of this strategy as a template for starting off your week strong. You can add, take away, and tweak to your heart's content. Make it your own. Once you get into a groove, you'll be amazed at how meal prepping becomes second nature.

Getting Started

You'll need to set aside one day a week for a big shopping trip and to do a couple of hours of batch cooking. If you can, pick a day when you don't have to work. If you have the weekend off, Sunday works well. You can grocery shop the day before or in the morning of your meal-prep day. With enough planning you'll be able to create meals for Monday through Wednesday. On Thursday, a quick trip to the market and a mini meal-prep session will get you through the weekend. Adjust according to your day(s) off.

Must-Have Tools

I'm all about keeping it basic and buying tools that can multitask. Here's what I recommend for getting your meal prep on, the need-to-haves:

- Programmable slow cooker or Instant Pot electronic pressure cooker
- Blender for sauces and soups
- Sharp chef's knife and paring knife for prep work
- Cutting boards—one for veggies and one for meat
- Baking sheets for roasting tons of veggies
- Large cast-iron skillet for stovetop-to-oven dishes
- Simple set of pots and pans—stainless steel is a good bet
- Lots of glass-lock containers to store all your tasty eats

In addition, here are some nice-to-haves you may want to add to your quiver:

- Microplane grater for zesting citrus and grating ginger or garlic
- Julienne peeler or spiralizer for making veggie noodles
- Dutch oven to braise the most scrumptious, fall-apart-tender roasts

Meal-Prep Strategy

Find Your Framework

For a meal-prep strategy that's structured but gives you plenty of options, think of cooking different types of dishes. For example, you might make a soup or stew, a slow-cooked protein, a couple of trays of roasted veggies, etc. That framework means you're not constantly guessing, but you're free to mix up the actual recipes and keep it interesting. Once you dial in your framework, it's smooth sailing.

Here are some suggestions to inspire you:

Hard-boil a batch of eggs (great for a quick snack).

Roast a couple of trays of chopped veggies.

Prepare a soup or stew, which freezes well.

Make a frittata or egg muffins (great portable breakfasts).

Slow-cook a roast, chicken, or other chunk of protein.

Fry up some burgers.

Make a sauce or two—salsa, guacamole, homemade balsamic vinaigrette, homemade mayo, and chimichurri are some of my favorites.

Roast a half dozen sweet potatoes or white potatoes.

Blend up a batch of homemade nut milk.

Make some chia pudding or overnight oats for a fast breakfast.

Chop up some bags of fresh veggies for quick cooking later in the week.

Cook a big batch of bone broth.

Experiment and find your best mix!

Use All Your Cooking Tools

Work smarter, not harder. Spread the work around your kitchen by making use of all your cooking tools. For example, baking everything means you'll have a lot of lag time as you wait. An efficient meal-prep session means using all your resources so there's no downtime. You'll finish faster if you put something in the slow cooker and make use of the oven while something else is simmering away on the stovetop.

Roll Food Forward

Once you get more comfortable with meal prepping, it'll be easier to roll food forward. That means repurposing leftovers in other meals. Maybe you roast a couple of chickens on your meal-prep day and pull the meat off. One evening you serve the meat from one chicken at dinner along with some roasted veggies, while the meat from the other becomes a chicken salad for your lunches. Then you put the bones in your slow cooker or Instant Pot and cook up a nourishing batch of broth. Two birds, one stone. (Couldn't resist the pun!)

Add a Sauce or Spice It Up

Seasoning your meal-prep proteins and veggies very simply with salt and pepper means they're a blank canvas you can spice or sauce up later to keep it fresh. For example, toss some meatballs with basil, garlic, and tomato sauce one day. The next day, chop up the rest of the batch and add it to a southwestern omelet with chili powder and salsa.

Double It!

If you're going to use the oven to roast one tray of veggies, maximize the space and roast two! Double up on your favorite soups and stews—those freeze well—and make some deposits to your freezer food bank.

Clean as You Go

You know what nobody loves about meal prep? Staring down Dish Mountain at the end. To keep things manageable, clean a little as you go. Wash your cutting board, pots, and pans between recipes. Enlist family to dry dishes. And for heaven's sake, use parchment paper on your baking trays for nonstick roasting and easy cleanup. It's the little things!

The Non-Breakfast Breakfast and "Brinner"

You can do anything you want! That means you can eat breakfast for dinner or dinner for breakfast. The first meal of the day does not have to be a traditional sweet dish like cereal or pastries. Try something outside the box. My favorite breakfast food is home-made soup—warm, nourishing, and satisfying.

Try a Meal Exchange

Rope a couple of friends into a meal exchange: Cook and prepare a main dish, side dish, and sauce for your friends and yourself. Swap portions, and you have instant variety!

Include Pantry Staples

- Canned or bottled diced tomatoes and green chilies (great for quick stews and sauces)
- Tuna, sardines, and smoked oysters (instant no-cook, nutrient-dense protein)

- Prepared salsas (add flavor to just about everything)

- Coconut milk (curry in a hurry, coming right up)

- Coconut aminos or gluten-free tamari (soy sauce substitutes)

- Low-sodium chicken or vegetable broth (forms the base of any quick soup)

- Dried mushrooms (rehydrate and add to soups, frittatas, or rice for an instant umami flavor)

- Ghee or olive, avocado, or coconut oils (for cooking and drizzling)

- Vinegar (I like apple cider and balsamic for quick dressings)

- Herbs and spices (a few of my faves: garlic powder, smoked paprika, cumin, thyme, and dill)

CREATE YOUR CORE 4 PLEDGE

Another thing: this program isn't pass or fail. Once you commit to it, stay with it. If you eat, drink, think, or do something you regret, stay grounded in the present. You did it. It's over and done with. Resolve to try your best going forward and move the heck on. You don't have to go back to Day 1 and start over again. If you miss a day, simply keep going the next day. In other words, life is lived in the gray areas.

I also encourage you to create a pledge to underscore your resolve—now, while you're motivated and excited. Here's mine: "Every day I'll do my best to nourish, strengthen, and energize my body. I'll do my best to stay in the present, and I'll hold nobody but myself accountable for my actions. Most of all, I'll make an effort to treat myself with kindness and compassion."

You can adopt this pledge as your own or think of a few sentences that will guide you and keep you centered on this journey. Keep it focused on the positive, on what you want to do. Once you've created your pledge, write it on three small pieces of paper and post them in different places where you'll see it daily (like your bathroom mirror, nightstand, and work station).

COMPLETE THE CORE 4 HEALTH TRACKER

In the Pillar 4 chapter you created your Personal Pillar Plan, where you identified your priorities and clarified what you want to improve. The Personal Pillar Plan also helps you check your progress later in the program. At the end of this chapter you'll fill out a Health Tracker, a yardstick for measuring how specific aspects of your life and health change during the program. You have to know where you're starting from when you begin the program; otherwise, at the end, how will you really know if something changed? (The human memory is notoriously fuzzy.)

The Health Tracker is a broad assessment; you'll consider physical, mental, and emotional factors, such as "How my clothes fit compared to when I felt at my best," "My attitude toward exercise," and "How adaptable and flexible I am." You'll rank more than forty dimensions of your health on a scale of one to ten at the beginning of the program as well as at the end, for evidence of how you've changed.

If you're a quantitative person and you really need to see more details of your progress, the best thing you can do is a dual-energy x-ray absorptiometry (DEXA) scan, which accurately measures your body composition and bone density. Or take measurements of yourself before and after so you'll have evidence of how you've changed physically. I don't recommend weighing yourself. Remember, this journey is about gaining health, and the scale cannot accurately reflect changes in your body composition, your thinking, or your energy levels.

NEXT UP: BECOME THE BEST VERSION OF YOU

I want to take a moment and acknowledge you for taking action and preparing for the program. You're here. You're ready. And you deserve to be the best version of you that you're envisioning. Repeat that: "I deserve to be the best version of me that I'm envisioning."

Feel it in your gut. Feel it in your heart.

That's powerful energy.

Knowledge without action doesn't get results. As you move through each day, you'll develop a set of tools to carry with you . . . for life. You'll be well equipped to make lasting change!

Health Tracker

Do this assessment at the beginning and at the end of the program. The goal is to reflect on how other metrics of health and well-being—other than the scale—have changed. The directions are quite simple. Rank your current assessment of each dimension on a scale of 1 to 10 (1 is the lowest; 10 is the highest).

	Day 1 *Date*	Day 31 *Date*
How my clothes fit now compared to when I felt at my best	_____	_____
How I feel about the quality of the food I eat	_____	_____
How I feel about my relationship with food	_____	_____
How often I use diets to control my eating habits	_____	_____
How I feel about the types of food choices I make on a daily basis	_____	_____
The quality of my sleep on average	_____	_____
The number of hours I sleep on average	_____	_____
How rested I feel in the morning	_____	_____
How easy it is to start my day	_____	_____
How I feel about my stress level	_____	_____
How resilient I feel after stressful events	_____	_____
How easy it is for me to relax	_____	_____
How happy I feel on average	_____	_____
The quality of my skin, hair, and nails	_____	_____
The quality of my digestion	_____	_____
How good my mood is on a daily basis	_____	_____
How confident I feel about my abilities	_____	_____
How confident I feel about my appearance	_____	_____
How often I speak or think poorly about myself or think degrading thoughts	_____	_____

How often I let stories from my past keep me stuck in the present   ____   ____

How often I get insatiable food cravings   ____   ____

How clear my mind is, instead of foggy   ____   ____

How much energy I have throughout the day   ____   ____

How much I rely on caffeine or sugar to get through my day   ____   ____

How often I take renewing breaks throughout the day   ____   ____

How addicted I am to social media   ____   ____

How sedentary I am on an average day, excluding exercise   ____   ____

My motivation to exercise   ____   ____

My attitude toward exercise   ____   ____

My overall strength level   ____   ____

My stamina during exercise   ____   ____

My satisfaction with my career   ____   ____

How stressed I feel at work   ____   ____

How valued I feel at work   ____   ____

How stressed I feel about money   ____   ____

How clear my sense of purpose in this world is   ____   ____

My satisfaction with the most important relationships in my life   ____   ____

How adaptable and flexible I am   ____   ____

How easy it is for me to complete something even if I'm not
really excited about it   ____   ____

How often I make specific outcome-focused goals
(such as lose 10 pounds or pay off a debt)   ____   ____

How satisfied I am with my current body composition
(body fat and muscle)   ____   ____

How good I feel overall   ____   ____

Before you begin the 30-day program, answer the following questions based on your Health Tracker answers:

Pick five things you ranked low (under 5). Write them below:

_____

_____

_____

_____

_____

Think of the Core 4 pillars—Eat Nourishing Foods, Move with Intention, Recharge Your Energy, Empower Your Mind. Which pillar(s) do you recognize need to be built and balanced the most in your life?

_____

_____

_____

_____

_____

Imagine yourself a year from now. Describe what your life will feel like. Really express your greatest desires for yourself . . . nobody is going to see this except for you. Talk about the things you'll be feeling and doing. Hold nothing back. Now is your chance to dream big.

_____

_____

_____

_____

_____

Kick It Off

You've had a chance to wrap your brain around the guiding framework of the Core 4 program. Now it's time to take action. Unlike some plans that focus on one element of health (diet or fitness), during each week you'll dabble in each of the Core 4 pillars. Every day will include a lesson and a challenge.

DAY 0: MEAL-PREP DAY

One of the most common worries about starting the Core 4 isn't working out, going to bed earlier, or even exercising . . . it's what to eat! And rightly so, considering that eating is something we do multiple times a day. Maybe you don't have a lot of experience in the kitchen or you're a little rusty. Maybe learning this nutrient-dense way of eating means your old standby meals need some tweaking. Whatever it is, I've got you.

At the start of each week you'll see a suggested meal-prep framework that will guide you through the whole program. As written, the meal plan usually feeds one or two people. If you're new to cooking, these meal plans will help you create some structure and guidance so you're not rushing at the last minute to prepare every meal fresh.

As I mentioned in the previous chapter, included in each week are two meal-prep days—one large and one small—with recipes from "The Core 4 Recipes" chapter (page 255) plus a few other simple staples to prepare, like roasting veggies and hard-boiling eggs. I recommend grocery shopping the day before, but do what makes the most sense for you. The idea is that you'll make a bunch of food ahead of time so all you have to do is reheat and eat. I give most leftovers three to five days in the refrigerator, as long as they're properly stored in airtight containers—I recommend glass-lock containers with snap-on lids. Not going through the food as fast as you thought? Most dishes are freezable for at least a month, often far longer, so pop the extra servings in cold storage for later.

During this first week try to follow the meal plan as written. In the weeks that follow you'll naturally figure out ways to tweak the plans to suit you. Take into account your best food prep days, your appetite, your food preferences, and any food restrictions you're dealing with. The more you can make meal preparation your own, the more likely you are to stick to the program. And remember, any dish can be breakfast!

Week 1 Shopping List

Bacon (16 ounces)
Deli ham, high quality
    (24 slices)
Eggs (3 dozen)
Ground pork (8 ounces)
Ground turkey breast
    (2 pounds)
Pork shoulder roast
    (3 to 4 pounds)
Shrimp (8 ounces)

Blueberries (2 cups)
Broccoli (2 pounds)
Butter lettuce (1), optional
Carrots (3 pounds)
Cauliflower (2 pounds)

Cherry tomatoes (12)
Cucumber (1), optional
Dill (1 bunch)
Green cabbage (1), optional
Green onions (2) + Green
    onion (1), optional
Herbs, fresh (mint, cilantro,
    Thai basil—for pho
    meal), optional
Jalapeño pepper (1),
    optional
Lemon (1)
Lime (1) + Lime (1), optional
Mung bean sprouts
    (1 4-ounce package),
    optional

Oranges (2)
Parsley or mint (2 bunches)
Red onion (1)
Shallot (1)
Spinach
    (2 eight-ounce bags)
Sweet potatoes (3)
Tomato (1), optional
Yellow onion (1)
Zucchini (2 pounds)

Almonds (¼ cup)
Apple cider vinegar
    (2 tablespoons)
Apple juice, no sugar added
    (4 cups)

Beef broth, low-sodium (8 cups)

Black olives, pitted (¼ cup)

Butter, grass-fed and unsalted (2 tablespoons)

Cinnamon stick (1)

Cloves, whole (2)

Coconut aminos (1 tablespoon)

Extra-virgin olive oil or ghee

Fish sauce (1 tablespoon plus ¼ teaspoon)

Garlic powder (1 teaspoon)

Ginger, ground (¼ teaspoon)

Oregano, dried (1 teaspoon)

Peanuts, chopped (1 tablespoon), optional

Salsa, prepared (½ cup)

Red pepper flakes (⅛ teaspoon), optional

Rice noodles (1 8-ounce package) or zucchini (1 pound), optional

Salt and pepper

Sesame oil, dark (½ teaspoon)

Sesame seeds (1 teaspoon), optional

Sriracha or chili oil, optional

Star anise (3)

DAY 0: MEAL-PREP DAY

Meals to prep:

» Savory Ham and Egg Cups (page 259), double the recipe (save a few in the fridge for tomorrow and freeze the rest)

» Shrimp Yum Balls (page 283)

» Chopped Broccoli Salad (page 269)

» Greek Turkey Burgers (page 282)

Other prep:

» 3 sweet potatoes, roast

» 1 bag fresh spinach, steam

» 12 eggs, hard-boil

» 8 ounces bacon, bake

» 2 pounds cauliflower, roast

DAY 1

BREAKFAST: Hard-boiled eggs + bacon + steamed spinach

LUNCH: Greek Turkey Burgers + Chopped Broccoli Salad

DINNER: Shrimp Yum Balls + roasted sweet potato

DAY 2

BREAKFAST: Savory Ham and Egg Cups + roasted cauliflower

LUNCH: Shrimp Yum Balls + steamed spinach

DINNER: Greek Turkey Burgers + Chopped Broccoli Salad

DAY 3

BREAKFAST: Hard-boiled eggs + bacon + roasted sweet potato

LUNCH: Greek Turkey Burgers + Chopped Broccoli Salad

DINNER: Shrimp Yum Balls + roasted cauliflower

DAY 4

BREAKFAST: Hard-boiled eggs + roasted sweet potato + steamed spinach

LUNCH: Savory Ham and Egg Cups + roasted cauliflower

DINNER: Apple Braised Pork Shoulder (prepare today) + Roasted Carrots with Orange Dill Butter (prepare today)

Meals to prep:

» Apple Braised Pork Shoulder (page 279)

» Fast Weeknight Pho (page 265)

» Roasted Carrots with Orange Dill Butter (page 270)

Other prep:

» 2 pounds zucchini, roast

DAY 5

BREAKFAST: Hard-boiled eggs + bacon + roasted zucchini

LUNCH: Fast Weeknight Pho

DINNER: Apple Braised Pork Shoulder + Roasted Carrots with Orange Dill Butter

DAY 6

BREAKFAST: Savory Ham and Egg Cups + Roasted Carrots with Orange Dill Butter

LUNCH: Apple Braised Pork Shoulder + roasted zucchini

DINNER: Fast Weeknight Pho

DAY 1: MOVEMENT

Welcome to Day 1. Today's a big day. It's the beginning of the Core 4 program and the start of a new phase of your life, one in which you'll start unlearning the shit that's not serving you and move into a bolder, bigger way of nourishing and strengthening yourself. Hopefully you're following along with Week 1's nutrition plan, which means you've already prepped meals today like a boss. But we're not going to talk about food quiiiite yet. Instead, I want to ask you a very important question: How much time do you spend sitting?

Even if you exercise regularly, you may be living a sedentary life. In today's world, it's become easier to do less and less—and a body that is not in motion tends to remain not in motion. (Oh, that Isaac Newton. What a guy!)

Movement is more than exercise—it includes all the activity you do throughout a day. And if you're like most people, you probably spend most of your day sitting. That can have a huge effect on everything from how much energy you use to how stiff and immobile you feel.

While the news is full of headlines like SITTING IS THE NEW SMOKING, I don't want to skip right to sensationalism. And let's certainly not have a heap of guilt if we sit a lot. Remember, action is what matters most.

It's very common for someone who works out to still be sedentary the rest of the day. It's really not our fault: Remember that thing where our environment and our biology are mismatched? It applies here too. We commute to work, sit at our jobs for hours on end (thanks to antiquated corporate culture), commute home, and then collapse exhausted on the couch.

If you took a trip down history lane, you'd find our ancestors hunting and gathering. There was a lot of low-level physical work to be done daily. And certainly, when the hunt was on, there was a big burst of intense activity followed by recovery. Even in

more modern agricultural times, there was plenty of labor to be done. You may have a job that demands physical activity—nurse, military worker, or household CEO—but our modern society has phased out a lot of labor. The difference between then and now is that low level of baseline activity. Think chores, walking, taking care of the house, and preparing food.

So if you're currently pretty sedentary, even if you work out regularly, what can you do about it? The answer isn't to exercise more; it's to incorporate more NEPA: non-exercise physical activity—all the other movement you do besides your dedicated workout. (We covered this in detail along with NEAT in the Pillar 2 chapter, so if you need a refresher, head to page 52.)

To put it simply, the more you move each day, the more calories you burn. The rad part about this type of activity is that it's low-intensity and doesn't require recovery time. And it doesn't usually come with the associated increase in appetite that intense workouts do.

NEPA can amount to several hundred calories burned each day! Examples include

- Light housework
- Walking
- Doing errands
- Cooking
- Gardening
- Playing with the kids
- Getting up from your desk frequently . . . every half-hour, for example
- Parking farther away from your destination and walking
- Fidgeting and constantly changing position
- Light stretching

Compare these two stories:

SANDRA A: Sandra wakes up ten minutes before she needs to leave for work and eats an energy bar for breakfast while on her forty-five-minute commute on the

train to work. She's a financial analyst at a big firm and spends most of her day in meetings or at her computer. At lunch, she usually grabs something from the work cafeteria and spends the rest of her break answering emails.

She's out the door at 5:00 p.m. and spends another forty-five minutes on the train. Once she gets home, she orders dinner in and watches a few hours of TV before bed. Three times a week she goes to a fitness class at a local gym.

SANDRA B: Sandra wakes up forty-five minutes before leaving for work each day. She cooks herself a simple breakfast or warms up leftovers and empties the dishwasher before she heads out. She commutes forty-five minutes on the train to work, but she gets off one stop early to add a few blocks of walking. She's a financial analyst at a big firm and spends most of her day in meetings or at her computer.

Recently, she switched to a standing desk and has set an alarm to alert her every thirty minutes, when she walks to fill her water bottle or does some simple stretches, like side bends and shoulder rolls. At lunch, she usually walks a few streets away to grab something at a local deli. She's out the door at 5:00 pm, walks a few blocks to the train, and spends forty-five minutes commuting home. She often stands for short periods.

Once she gets home, Sandra cooks a simple dinner. Sometimes she watches a show, then she does other chores before bed, tidies up, and lays out her clothes for the next day. Three times a week she goes to a fitness class at a local gym.

Clearly, Sandra B has more movement in her day.

Why did I give you a tale of two Sandras? Because I know that you can't always switch from commuting to your job and working in an office to something else. What you *can* do is look for more opportunities within your daily structure to move more often.

Move Your Body

This week is all about getting in touch with basic movement, so there won't be any exercises with weights. Even if you're conditioned to exercising already, I want you to do these movements without weights. Take your time and move through the sets, listening to your body and resting as needed.

Once you're past the warm-up, complete all the sets of each movement before moving on to the next. Both levels 1 and 2 should perform this week's workouts. If you move with intention, the exercises will help pinpoint areas where you may need to work more—like your mobility, stability, or flexibility.

Day 1 Challenge: Work Out

Remember to respect your body! Don't do anything that causes pain.

WRIST WARM-UP SEQUENCE—*2 sets*

Stand with your arms in front of you at waist height. Roll your wrists around in circles in both directions, then use your left hand to gently stretch your right hand forward, backward, and from side to side to stretch your wrist. Repeat the actions with the left hand.

CAT COWS—*3 sets of 6 reps*

Get on your hands and knees with your hands under your shoulders and knees under your hips. Keep your neck neutral as you look at the floor. Breathe in as you lift your head and let your belly soften. Then exhale as you curl your back up like a cat and lower your head. Repeat, moving slowly and experiencing the stretch through your shoulders and neck.

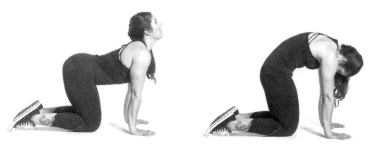

INCHWORMS—*2 sets of 50 feet*

Stand with your feet under your hips. Hinge at the waist and put your hands on the floor in front of you. Engage your core and walk your hands out a few inches, keeping your legs straight. Then walk your feet toward your hands, using small steps. Repeat, "inching" along the floor.

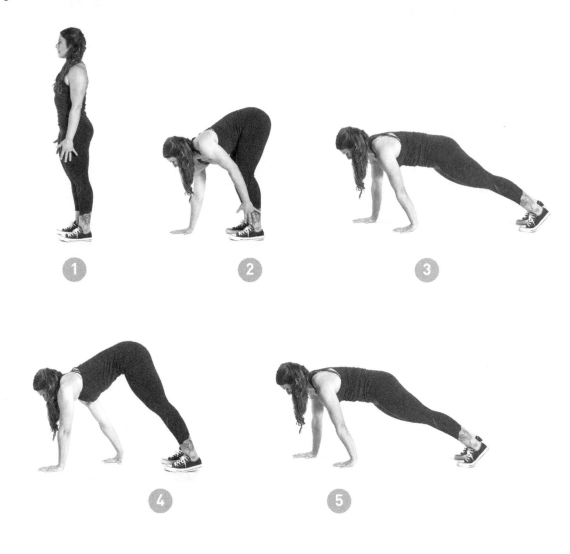

SINGLE-LEG STANDING BALANCES—*4 sets on each leg*

Stand with your feet under your hips. Shift your weight onto your left leg and slowly lift your right foot off the floor until your knee makes a 90-degree angle. Extend your arms for balance. Hold for 10 to 30 seconds, then lower the right foot and repeat on the other side, lifting your left leg. Note that doing this move barefoot will let you grip the floor and balance more easily.

HIP HINGES WITH STICK—*3 sets of 8 reps*

Stand with your feet under your hips while holding a broomstick or PVC pipe against your spine, with one hand at the back of your neck and one hand at your lower back. Keep your legs straight as you slowly shift your weight back and fold at your hips to bring your head toward the floor. Keep the broomstick against the back of your head, upper back, and butt. Then return to a standing position.

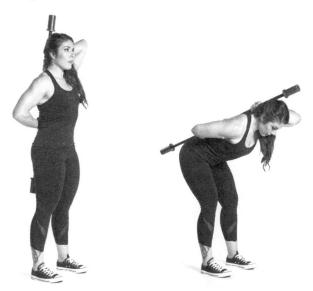

SQUATS—*3 sets of 10 reps*

Stand with your feet under your hips. Keeping your feet flat on the floor, engage your core as you push your hips back and bend your knees, lowering until your thighs are a little lower than parallel to the floor (or as low as feels comfortable). Go as low as you can while keeping a neutral spine. Your knees should track over your feet, and your chest should remain up. Then return to the starting position.

DAY 2: GUT CHECK

Yesterday you did your first challenge. Frickin' awesome! Sometimes the hardest part is getting started and creating some forward momentum. Let's keep it going.

If you're a little sore, that's normal. Challenging your muscles to move in new ways shakes things up! Taking a short walk or doing some light yoga can help ease any soreness. With Day 1 and some movement in the books, now you'll turn your eye inward to matters of the mind.

Your brain is capable of so many amazing feats. Planning, language, movement, and gathering sensory information are mostly tasks of the outermost brain layer, called the cortex. If you use the analogy that your brain is like an onion, the outermost papery skin would be the cortex. But deeper in the brain, in the innermost core of the onion, is another cluster of structures: the limbic brain. I don't want to turn this into an anatomy lesson, but this will help you understand why you have "gut" feelings.

The limbic brain is a collection of structures that include the hypothalamus and the amygdala, which generates feelings, emotions, and primal urges. Now here's the kicker: the limbic brain can't produce language. That's the reason why we struggle to put our gut feelings or intuition into words. Whether we feel a decision in our gut or our heart, or it feels like intuition, it's really the limbic brain that's responsible. In his book *Start with Why*, Simon Sinek writes:

> Our limbic brain is powerful, powerful enough to drive behavior that sometimes contradicts our rational and analytical understanding of a situation. We often trust our gut even if the decision flies in the face of all the facts and figures . . .

When you force people to make decisions with only the rational part of their brain, they almost invariably end up "overthinking" . . . In contrast, decisions made with the limbic brain, gut decisions, tend to be faster, higher-quality decisions.

If you've ever taken a multiple-choice test, you probably know this experience well. Often your first instinct—your gut feeling—about the answer is right. If you go back and mull it over, you may talk yourself out of the correct answer as you think harder and harder.

Tuning In to Your Gut

I don't want you to walk away with the impression that rational decision-making doesn't have a place in your life. But I do want you to consider times when your gut or intuition was telling you to do one thing and, after a period of agonizing over the decision, you went with the opposite choice.

How did it turn out? How easy was it to make the gut decision versus the rational decision?

More important, how many times have you ignored your gut because you wouldn't be able to justify your decision to someone else?

My hope is that this lesson will highlight the importance of listening to your gut and tuning in to how your body feels when you make decisions based on intuition. If a gut decision feels light, energetic, and good in your body, that's something to listen to. It might even feel a little "terrexcitifying" (to quote my friend Allegra).

On the other hand, if a decision feels heavy, dark, or bad in your body, there's merit in that too . . . even if you can't explain it in words.

Day 2 Challenge: Get in Touch with Your Gut

On a piece of paper or in a journal, complete the following prompts. It's important to write these down and get them out of your head:

When I feel stressed or worried, my body feels like . . .

When I go with my gut, my body feels like . . .

Write about a time you listened to your gut. Was the decision easy or hard to make? Why do you think that is?

DAY 3: CORE OF THE MATTER

Hopefully during yesterday's lesson on gut feelings you gained some clarity around how your body and brain talk to each other and which signs to feel for. Listening to your body isn't always easy, especially when the whole damn world wants you to be logical 24/7 and accuses women of being too emotional. Intuition is your superpower! Now let's see how to set the stage for continuing to build your physical strength.

The root of all safe and effective movement is posture and alignment. The clients I coach in the gym often spend half an hour or more each day mobilizing their bodies, rolling out stiff tissue, and trying to improve their flexibility. While these interventions have merit, it's hard to undo the effects of poor posture.

Think of how much time you spend sitting or standing each day. How you sit or stand outside of workout time can affect your ability to move effectively during your workout and how you move in general. You may slouch, creating rounded shoulders, a tucked pelvis, and a forward head position. All of these may lead to stiffness, discomfort, or even pain.

On the other hand, women are often taught to stick out their chests and bums, which can cause a hyperextension of the upper back and an anterior (forward) pelvic position, leading to back issues and pain. High heels often make that problem worse, putting a lot of pressure on the lumbar region, or lower back.

To correct your posture, stand with your feet under your hips and think about lightly squeezing your glutes, or butt muscles, to stop the pelvis from rolling forward. Then think about tucking your ribs by lightly engaging your upper abs—it's a bit of a strange sensation at first. This aligns your spine. With your hands at your sides, turn your palms up to the sky, then lower your hands. This keeps your shoulders from rolling forward and putting strain on your neck. The same general rules apply for sitting.

When you stand, it's also important to point your toes forward instead of in or out. This may take some practice, but again, it helps to better align your skeleton from the feet on up. You can also look for wear patterns on your shoes to see if you tend to stand toes out or in.

Chronic joint pain or muscular tension is often traced back to posture and how the feet are oriented. For example, standing duck-footed, with the toes out, can cause the arches to collapse, which can make your inner knees sag toward each other.

Changing postural habits takes time, but it's worth the investment to start improving your posture.

Now let's talk about strengthening your core. Make no mistake: having a strong and stable trunk is just as important as strengthening your arms and legs. And if you plan to lift weights, it's even more imperative. Your core muscles involve far more than just the rectus abdominus—the abs that make a six-pack. They include the deeper abdominal muscle layers as well as your back muscles, glutes, diaphragm, and pelvic floor.

The good news is that the Core 4 workouts include accessory work to help improve your core stability. Movements like planks may be well known, but others, like rows and waiter walks, will help you build the complete package. Even exercises as simple as squats and deadlifts are excellent for strengthening your core muscles.

Day 3 Challenge: Work Out

Note that levels 1 and 2 both complete this workout. Complete all sets and reps of each movement before moving on to the next.

ANKLE WARM-UP—*2 sets*

In a standing position, lift your right heel off the floor. Do ten ankle circles clockwise, and ten counterclockwise. Repeat these movements with your left foot.

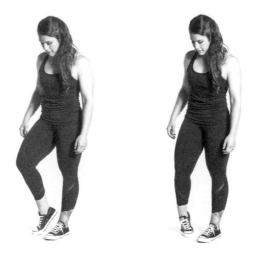

GLUTE BRIDGES—*3 sets of 10 reps*

Lie on your back with your knees bent, your feet flat on the floor and close to your hips, and your arms at your sides on the floor. Engage your core and squeeze your butt as you slowly drive your hips up toward the ceiling so that your body is in a straight line from head to knees. Keep your knees parallel to each other; don't let them collapse in or out. Slowly lower your hips back to the starting position.

Pro Tip

» *To make it harder,* lift up one leg at a time from the bridge position.

DOWN DOGS—*4 sets of holding for 10 seconds*

Start on your hands and knees, with your hands under your shoulders and your knees under your hips. Exhale as you straighten your legs and arms and push your hips up toward the ceiling to make an inverted V with your body. Actively drive your palms into the floor, and actively lift your sit bones toward the ceiling. Elongate through your spine, and keep your gaze on the floor ahead of you to maintain a neutral neck. Bend your knees to lower back down to the starting position.

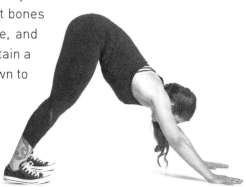

Pro Tip

» Use a yoga mat or carpet so your hands don't slip.

DUCK WALKS—*2 sets of 50 feet*

Stand with your feet under your hips, your arms at your sides. Turn your toes out slightly and engage your core. Push your hips back and bend your knees, lowering into a partial squat position. Slowly step forward, maintaining your squat position. Try to keep yourself from bouncing up and down as you walk.

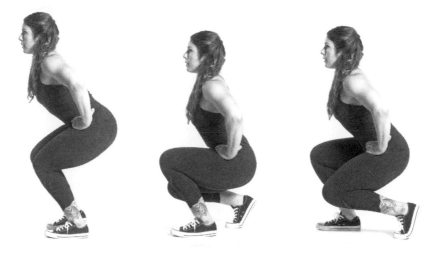

BEAR CRAWLS—*2 sets of 50 feet forward, 2 sets of 50 feet backward*

Start on your hands and knees. Slowly crawl forward with your knees off the ground. Keep your butt low instead of letting it stick up in the air, and try to keep from bouncing up and down. If your shoulders or arms tire, rest for a few seconds before continuing.

Pro Tip

» *To make it harder,* stay lower to the floor by bending your arms.

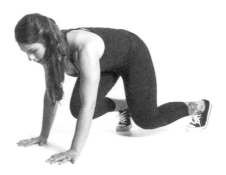

UPPER BACK TWISTS—*3 sets of 6 reps on each side*

Get on your hands and knees, with your hands under your shoulders and your knees under your hips. Shift your weight onto your left hand and bring your right arm under and across your body with the palm facing up. Keeping your hand there, slowly twist your upper body toward the ceiling. Then untwist, placing your right hand back on the floor. Repeat the movement with the opposite arm.

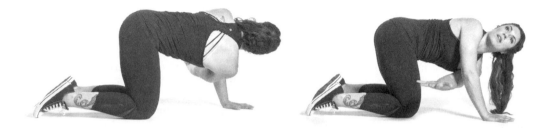

DAY 4: SLEEP, PART 1

So far, you've dabbled in three of the four pillars. Well done! Small actions add up, and you're experimenting with some different tools from your new health toolbox. Taking action is where it's at, so keep the momentum going. Now it's time to dive into one huge way you recharge your energy: sleep.

If you're already getting eight hours in a dark room, sleeping through the night, and waking well rested, you deserve my kudos. If I didn't just describe you, you've got some work to do. As you read in the Pillar 3 chapter, a chronic lack of sleep totally messes with your health, your energy levels, and your cravings, among other things.

My sleep habits weren't always great. I routinely ended the evening by falling asleep in front of the television, got less than six hours in bed, and slept in a room that had lots of ambient light. I was also training hard at the time, and my sleep habits hurt my physical and mental performance. As I mentioned before, somewhere between seven and nine hours of sleep is best, depending on the person.

If you're eating a pristine diet and working out a perfect amount but your sleep is a wreck, this is a huge area for improvement. It can be hard to change your sleep, but nutrition and moving your body can help. Later in the program, I'll give you some practical tips to implement so that you fall asleep faster and sleep more soundly. For now, pay attention to how much sleep you're getting and keep track of sleep disruptions.

Day 4 Challenge: For the Next Seven Days, Track Your Sleep

Note sleep and wake times. If you got up in the night to use the bathroom or couldn't fall back to sleep, note that too. Write down anything you think may be throwing a monkey wrench in your sleep, like eating a late dinner, reading a stressful email before bed, etc. An app like Sleep Cycle is a great way to get started. Or you can keep a log in the Notes app on your phone or in a journal. Looking at the bigger picture of a week can help you identify trends and patterns. If you can keep it going for more than a week, even better!

DAY 5: LIFT "HEAVY"

Yesterday you were reminded about the importance of sleep. If you're tempted to sacrifice Zs, remember that rest time isn't a luxury—it's a necessity for feeling primed and ready to kick ass every day. And you'll need that mental and physical energy to tackle today's challenge.

Getting stronger means (eventually) moving "heavy" shit. Long gone are the days when most of us physically labored from sun up to sun down, tending camp, foraging and hunting for food, and hauling water. Our modern age allows us to work behind desks, sit in offices, and drive in our cars for long commutes. Most of us don't work the way we used to, and we're not as robust as our ancestors.

Unless we mimic what they did by moving heavy things.

Remember that you have different types of muscle fibers that respond to different activities. You use mostly slow-twitch fibers for long, low-key slow stuff—like walking, putzing around the house, or even running a half marathon. These activities don't require much force. It's the fast-twitch fibers—of which there are a

few kinds—that respond with heavier loads. They're associated with powerful and explosive movements.

But why does it matter? What if you don't want to do explosive movements? Well, here's the catch: Not only is using your full catalog of muscles better for balance, strength, and coordination, it's better for your metabolism. That translates to better hormonal balance. And that means better health overall.

Scary Heavy vs. Effective Dose

What if heavy things scare you?

First, it's natural to fear what we don't understand. That's why I'm here to guide you.

Lifting "heavy" doesn't mean your eyeballs will pop out of your head while a stupid-massive bar is about to crush you. It does mean pushing yourself out of your comfort zone a little.

Everyone starts somewhere, but even my seventy-five-year-old mother-in-law can lift more than 2-pound dumbbells. Weights shouldn't be so heavy that you can't use good form to lift them, but they have to be heavy enough that it's a challenge. No going through the motions!

Even the level 1 workout includes some weight lifting, though since you'll be using challenging weights, you may need a little more recovery time.

You don't need to work out *more* to see positive changes. When you lift moderate to heavy weights, you don't need to do long, complicated workouts daily to see results. In our house, we love the "minimum effective dose"—in other words, the minimum we can get away with to build strength without spending all our free time at the gym.

Day 5 Challenge: Work Out

Note that levels 1 and 2 both complete this workout. Complete all sets and reps of each movement before moving on to the next.

Make sure to track your sleep today.

WINDMILLS—*3 sets of 6 reps on each side*

Stand with your feet slightly wider than hip width apart and with your arms extended out to your sides at shoulder height. Engage your core and twist your body to bring your right hand toward your left foot. Return to the starting position, upright, and then twist your body to the left, bringing your left hand toward your right foot. Return again to the starting position and repeat.

Pro Tip

» *To make this harder,* hold a light dumbbell in the hand that's overhead. Do all the reps on one side before switching the dumbbell to the other hand and doing the reps on the other side.

SCAPULAR WALL SLIDES—*3 sets of 10 reps*

Stand with your back, shoulders, and butt against a wall. Lift your arms so they're against the wall with your arms bent at about a 45-degree angle, with your knuckles against the wall. Keeping your arms against the wall and your rib cage down, slowly slide your arms up and straighten them into a V shape. Reach as far as you can without pulling away from the wall or flaring at your ribs. Continue to maintain contact with the wall while you slowly slide your arms back to the starting position.

PERFECT STRETCHES—*2 sets of 50 feet*

Start with feet under your hips and your hands at your sides. Shift your weight onto your right foot and hug your left knee up toward your chest with your hands. Let go of your knee, then step your left foot forward and lower your right knee gently to the floor in a low lunge. Bring your right hand to the floor close to your left foot and lift your left hand up toward the ceiling, rotating your torso as you do so. Then set your left hand down next to your left foot, straighten both legs, and lift your left toe. Lean back to stretch your left hamstring. Raise your torso, step back, and repeat the movements on the other side.

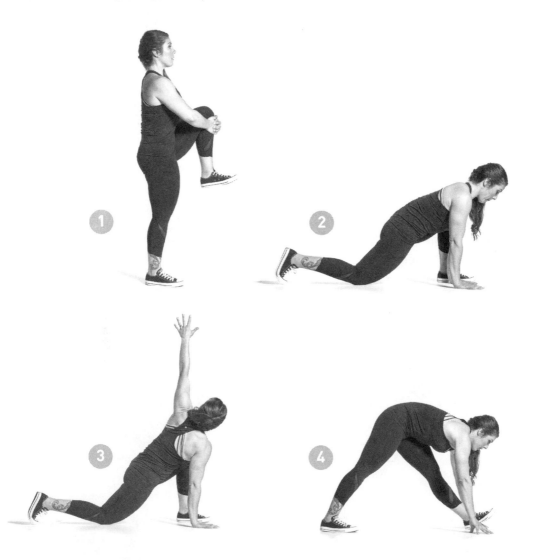

SPIDERMAN CRAWLS—*2 sets of 50 feet*

Start on your hands and knees, with your hands under your shoulders and your knees under your hips. Engage your core and reach your left hand forward, then place your left foot outside your left arm, bending your knee into a deep lunge. Keeping your body low, reach your right hand forward, followed by your right foot outside your right arm, bending your right knee. If you get tired, sit down and take a brief break, then resume.

Pro Tip

» *To make this harder,* take longer steps and stay very close to the floor.

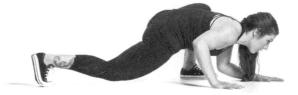

CRAB WALKS—*2 sets of 50 feet forward, 2 sets of 50 feet backward*

Sit with your knees bent and your feet flat on the floor. Push yourself up onto your hands and feet, with your hands under your shoulders and your feet hip width apart. "Walk" your hands and feet forward, keeping your butt low but off the floor. Try not to bounce your head and torso as you walk. If you get tired, sit down and take a brief break, then resume.

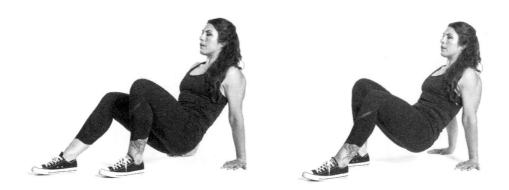

SQUATS—*3 sets of 10 reps*

Stand with your feet under your hips. Keeping your feet flat on the floor, engage your core as you push your hips back and bend your knees, lowering until your thighs are a little lower than parallel to the floor (or as low as feels comfortable). Go as low as you can while keeping a neutral spine. Your knees should track over your feet, and your chest should remain up. Then return to the starting position.

DAY 6: GOAL DIGGER

A little sore from yesterday's workout? That's good! It means you worked your muscles beyond what they're used to, and today you'll be repairing and rebuilding (aka getting stronger!) while you shift gears to think about your goals.

Motivational memes are everywhere these days. While it's great to see and reflect on them, they don't mean squat unless you have goals. Having goals, whether they're about eating or fitness or mindset, is key to keeping you working toward something and staying focused.

This is not to say that you have to be obsessed, which is counterproductive. But if you're drifting like a boat without a sail, it's time to establish some goals—as long as they're the right kind.

If your goals are too nebulous ("I want to save the rain forest") or are way too far from where you're at right now ("I'm going to squat 300 pounds," when your current is nowhere near that), they aren't serving you. Goals should be like little carrots dangling juuuuuuust beyond your grasp. They keep you reaching, striving, moving forward.

But having a goal isn't enough, even if it's detailed and specific. Think of the world's best duos:

Bacon and eggs

Han Solo and Chewbacca

Peanut butter and jelly

Squats and deadlifts

Like all dynamic pairs, your goals must be accompanied by action. If they're not, they sit on a shelf in your brain collecting cobwebs and dust.

The way to pump up the following goal-setting criteria is to add an action (or two or three) that says what you're going to *do*. You may have heard of SMART goals before. I like to make mine SMAART—the extra *A* stands for the *action* you'll take toward that goal.

What Makes a Goal SMAART?

A goal should be

> S = specific
> M = measurable
> A = achievable
> A = action driven
> R = realistic
> T = timely

What do SMAART goals look like? Check out the difference between these vague and SMAART goals:

> "I want to be healthier" versus "I'm going to include an extra veggie at each meal"

> "I want to get stronger" versus "I'm going to lift three times a week after work"

> "I want to be happier" versus "I'm going to take five minutes each day to write what I'm grateful for"

Outcome Focused Versus Process Focused

It's totally fine to have a final goal, an outcome that you want to reach. But it's often not the thing that will keep you moving forward and taking action. It can be hard to feel motivated when the target isn't close to your current reality. It's also hard to gauge your progress. Sometimes goals are so far away or so huge that your mind calls bullshit on you.

SMAART Goals Worksheet

Accountability matters. Until you write your goals out, they're just thoughts floating around in your head. Use this worksheet to write three concrete goals about any aspect of being healthy, happy, and more unbreakable. Remember to use the SMAART system:

Specific . . . Think of this like the what, where, when, why, and how of the goal.

Measurable . . . How will you measure your progress?

Achievable . . . Is the goal within reach but still challenging enough to make you stretch for it?

Action driven . . . Exactly which action are you going to take to make this happen?

Realistic . . . Are the goal and the timeframe realistic?

Timely . . . What's the timeframe? Open-ended goals with no timeframe are low on the motivational scale because there's no pressure at all.

Revisit your SMAART goals at the end of the program and rewrite them based on what you achieved!

Goal 1	Goal 2	Goal 3
S _____	S _____	S _____
M _____	M _____	M _____
A _____	A _____	A _____
A _____	A _____	A _____
R _____	R _____	R _____
T _____	T _____	T _____

Instead of focusing on the *outcome,* stay focused on the *process.*

What does that mean? Let's say your goal is to do ten pull-ups. If you can't even do one right now, that goal probably feels a bajillion miles away. There are so many factors that could go into your achieving even your first pull-up, and you can't predict exactly when everything is going to click.

On the other hand, let's say you commit every day to loosening up your tight shoulders with ten minutes of shoulder mobility and stretching. And every time you're in the gym, you practice increasing reps and sets of dumbbell rows and modified pull-ups to strengthen your upper body.

Which goal is going to feel more achievable and actionable? The latter.

You have direct control over doing your mobility and accessory exercises. That's something you can commit to and carry out. You'll keep getting stronger and eventually get your first pull-up. That'll lead to the next and, eventually, ten.

Day 6 Challenge: Complete the SMAART Goals Worksheet

After you complete the SMAART Goals Worksheet on page 129, jot your goals on three separate pieces of paper (sticky notes work well) and post those in three different places you see daily—in your car, on your fridge, in your training log, at work on your desk, etc.

Make sure to track your sleep today.

OPTIONAL WEEKEND WORKOUT. Remember Tabata interval training from the Pillar 2 chapter? It's fast! For this workout, do twenty seconds of squats, rest ten seconds, and repeat for eight rounds. Then tack on another Tabata set: push-ups for twenty seconds followed by ten seconds of rest, for eight rounds.

DAY 7: CRUSH CRAVINGS

How did you feel about setting your goals yesterday? That activity is often the kick in the pants you need to keep moving because you end up with a road map instead of just getting lost all the time. Today's challenge will help you crush your food cravings.

I'm going to be straight up here: The root causes of food cravings are diverse. And it isn't always possible to immediately stop them. But with consistency and healthy habits, you can minimize how often they rear their ugly heads.

Glad we got that out of the way. With that in mind, let's take a gander at some reasons you might be experiencing food cravings.

YOU'RE F'ING HUNGRY. I'm not trying to be flip here, but if you consistently eat tiny portions, your cravings might be actual hunger. Eat protein, carbs, and fat from real, whole foods at each meal in quantities that satiate your hunger for at least three to four hours. If you'd totally eat steamed fish and veggies right now, you're probably hungry.

YOUR GUT MICROBIOME NEEDS SUPPORT. Your gut is the site of many important biological functions, from food digestion and nutrient absorption to vitamin production to immunity. Your gut microbiome—the friendly bacteria that primarily live in your large intestine—plays a major role in keeping everything humming along. But sometimes these helpful gut bacteria overgrow in places they shouldn't or get displaced by harmful microbes. The causes may include poor diet, antibiotic overuse, stress, and incomplete digestion. This shift in the gut microbiome landscape can be associated with increased sugar cravings. Work with a qualified practitioner who can help identify the root issue and help you devise a plan for supporting your gut health.

YOU COULD HAVE LEPTIN RESISTANCE. Leptin is a hormone that communicates with the body about how much body fat you have. Leptin, much like insulin, can spike when you have less-than-optimal habits, like a diet high in processed food and poor sleep. Over time your body can become less capable of hearing the leptin signal. The best way to turn the boat around is to eat protein, carbs, and fat from real, whole foods and sleep eight or more hours a night.

YOUR CRAVINGS ARE STRESS RELATED. Very often cravings happen for completely non-food-related reasons. Stress is a big culprit. If you find yourself reaching for sweet, salty, fatty, or crunchy foods when you're stressed, create an interrupter habit that takes your mind off food and gets you out of the kitchen. You might decide that when stress-related cravings hit, you go take a walk around the block, fold some clothes, or write in your journal. If you're still hungry thirty minutes later, eat a healthy snack with protein, carbs, and fat.

IT'S THAT TIME OF THE MONTH. Shifts between estrogen and progesterone can amplify food cravings, specifically when estrogen is lower and progesterone is higher.

Protein Leverage

Protein leverage is an interesting hypothesis that makes a lot of sense, at least anecdotally. The idea is that if the food people eat is lacking in protein, they'll continue to eat whatever is around until they've reached a natural stopping point of about 15 percent of their calories from protein.

If the food around is low-nutrient, high-calorie ("empty") carbs and fats from processed food, a person would have to consume far too many calories in order to reach the protein threshold.

While this is still a hypothesis that requires further testing, it does seem to explain what people experience when their diet is low in protein, including a diet heavy in processed foods.

Personally, if I don't get a good whack of protein at breakfast, I often experience increased hunger and sometimes cravings throughout the day. Plus, if I fall behind on my protein intake at breakfast, it's hard to "make up" as the day goes on, because as a macronutrient, protein is the most satiating.

What does this mean for you? If you find yourself consistently hungry within one to two hours of eating a meal, check in with your protein intake. Whole food sources of protein from meat, seafood, and eggs are your most nutrient-dense options. You may need to bump up your protein intake slightly to find the level that works for your body. (Hint: It's often more than you'd think.)

Normally, estrogen drops after ovulation and progesterone rises; this helps explain why your appetite and cravings may be higher in the second half of your menstrual cycle. If you're in perimenopause, you may be experiencing wildly fluctuating hormone levels, and if you're in menopause, you're likely to be experiencing very low estrogen levels. All can contribute to cravings.

Day 7 Challenge: Prep Meals for Next Week

See the beginning of the next chapter for the upcoming week's shopping list and what to prep.

Make sure to track your sleep today.

WEEK 2

Settle In

You shook things up last week and took action. That takes courage and follow-through. Bravo!

I've gotta say, sometimes the first week is the toughest, so well done for sticking with it. You're making an effort to eat more mindfully and move in new ways, so it's totally normal for your body to start protesting like a cranky teenager who just had her electronics taken away—especially if you cut way back on sugar and processed food.

This too shall pass. As you head into Week 2, any low energy, headaches, and poor mood should start to lift. Doing things that are worthwhile isn't always easy, but you're strong AF, and I believe in you. If you still feel a little sluggish or sore this week, be sure you're well hydrated, getting enough sleep, and eating balanced meals. Don't underestimate the power of an evening walk (yay for more movement!), ten minutes of quiet time, or a little extra self-compassion. If flickers of doubt cross your mind, revisit your Core 4 Pledge (page 100).

Week 2 is when most people start settling in and feeling more comfortable with the Core 4, so let's go!

Week 2 Shopping List

Chicken breast (2 pounds)

Chicken sausage, any flavor
(1½ pounds)

Eggs (1 dozen)

Goat cheese, soft
(4 ounces), optional

Ground beef (1½ pounds)

Italian chicken sausage
(8 ounces)

Whole chicken
(3 to 4 pounds)

Beets (2)

Broccoli (1 pound)

Carrots (3)

Cauliflower (2 pounds)

Cilantro, fresh (1 bunch)

Ginger, fresh (1 inch)

Mint, fresh (1 bunch)

Parsley, fresh (1 bunch)

Garlic (2 heads)

Kale (2 bunches)

Lemons (2)

Parsnips (3)

Pear (1)

Red bell pepper (1)

Roma tomatoes (2)

Spinach (2 8-ounce bags)

Strawberries (1 pint),
optional

Sweet potatoes (3)

Yellow onions (4)

White potatoes (2)

Almond milk (2 cups)

Balsamic vinegar (¼ cup)

Basil, dried (2 teaspoons)

Chia seeds (5 tablespoons)

Chipotle pepper, ground
(½ teaspoon)

Coconut milk (16 ounces)

Collagen powder
(2 tablespoons), optional

Coriander, ground
(2 teaspoons)

Cumin, ground
(2 teaspoons)

Currants, dried, or raisins
(2 tablespoons)

Dijon mustard (1 teaspoon)

Extra-virgin olive oil or ghee

Fish sauce (1 teaspoon),
optional

Garam masala
(2 teaspoons)

Garlic powder (1 teaspoon)

Harissa sauce, mild
(2 tablespoons)

Honey (1 tablespoon),
optional

Parsley, dried (3 teaspoons)

Peanut butter, smooth
(¼ cup)

Peanuts or almonds,
chopped (2 tablespoons),
optional

Pecans (⅓ cup)

Pistachios, shelled (¼ cup)

Salt and pepper

Smoked paprika
(½ teaspoon)

Strawberries, frozen
(12 ounces)

Sun-dried tomatoes
(3 ounces)

Tahini (1 tablespoon)

Thyme, dried (1 teaspoon)

Tomato sauce (14 ounces)

Turmeric, ground
(2 teaspoons)

DAY 7

For this day's breakfast, lunch, and dinner, eat leftovers from the previous week.

Meals to prep:

- » Italian Frittata (page 258)

- » Chicken Tikka Masala (page 280)

- » Spinach, Pear, and Pecan Salad with Balsamic Vinaigrette (page 268), dressing stored on the side

- » Roasted Root Veggies (page 274)

Other prep:

- » 2 white potatoes, roast

- » 2 bunches fresh kale, steam

- » 1½ pounds chicken sausage, cook

DAY 8

BREAKFAST: Italian Frittata + steamed kale

LUNCH: Chicken sausage + Spinach, Pear, and Pecan Salad with Balsamic Vinaigrette

DINNER: Chicken Tikka Masala + roasted white potato

DAY 9

BREAKFAST: Italian Frittata + Roasted Root Veggies

LUNCH: Chicken Tikka Masala + roasted white potato

DINNER: Chicken sausage + Spinach, Pear, and Pecan Salad with Balsamic Vinaigrette

DAY 10

BREAKFAST: Savory Ham and Egg Cups + steamed kale

LUNCH: Italian Frittata + Spinach, Pear, and Pecan Salad with Balsamic Vinaigrette

DINNER: Chicken Tikka Masala + Roasted Root Veggies

DAY 11

BREAKFAST: Chicken sausage + Roasted Root Veggies

LUNCH: Italian Frittata + steamed kale

DINNER: Mini Meatloaf Sheet Tray Bake (prepare today)

Meals to prep:

» Mini Meatloaf Sheet Tray Bake (page 277)

» The Best Cauliflower Ever (page 273)

» PB and J Chia Breakfast Cups (page 261)

Other prep:

» 1 8-ounce bag fresh spinach, wash

» 1 chicken, roast

DAY 12

BREAKFAST: PB and J Chia Breakfast Cups + fresh spinach with olive oil and lemon juice

LUNCH: Shredded Chicken + The Best Cauliflower Ever

DINNER: Mini Meatloaf Sheet Tray Bake

DAY 13

BREAKFAST: PB and J Chia Breakfast Cups + fresh spinach with olive oil and lemon juice

LUNCH: Mini Meatloaf Sheet Tray Bake

DINNER: Shredded Chicken + The Best Cauliflower Ever

DAY 8: STRONG LEGS

Congrats on making it through the first week. How are you feeling? Was meal prep a little simpler yesterday than the first time you did it? Today I'm going to put my teach-

er's hat on for a bit and delve into the "why" of your workouts, specifically the reasons why strengthening your legs is important:

IT HELPS STRENGTHEN YOUR WHOLE BODY. When you weight train and use your leg muscles, you also use your core, or trunk, to stabilize the weights plus your arms to support the weights themselves. The result is more bang for your buck—you work out smarter, not longer.

YOU USE BIGGER MUSCLES. The major muscles of your legs—your quadriceps, hamstrings, and glutes—are bigger than your upper body muscles. By training these muscles, you're working more muscle fibers, and working more muscle fibers (the fast-twitch kind) means your body's ability to burn fat increases.

IT BUILDS YOUR MENTAL STRENGTH AND CONFIDENCE. A lot of fitness pros spend time teaching about the physical side of strengthening your legs but never the mental side of it. Squats, lunges, deadlifts, and carries aren't exactly easy. The mental fortitude it takes to complete your workout improves your ability to focus. And when you get physically stronger, achieving things you once thought impossible, your confidence soars and spills over into other aspects of your life.

These are just a few of the compelling reasons to strengthen your legs.

Functional Movement

Since you've completed the first week of movement, you've gotten a taste of the exercises I have planned for the remaining three weeks. These movements are by and large *functional* movements. That means they take you through natural, real-world, multi-joint ways of moving. For example, you squat every single day without thinking about it. When? Every time you sit down at your desk or use the toilet. And every time you reach up into a high cabinet to store something or put luggage into an overhead bin, that's a press. When's the last time you picked up a heavy bag of pet food or a heaped-up laundry basket? That's a deadlift.

When you spend most of your workout time focusing on functional movements, you

work multiple muscles at one time;

improve the efficiency of your workout;

promote better balance and coordination;

boost your metabolism;

improve hormonal balance; and

strengthen your body in ways that directly carry over to sports—and everyday life.

This is why I don't use machines in the Core 4 program. Let's say you're doing leg presses on a machine. You lie passively on a sturdy surface and push with your legs. Your body isn't doing as much to maintain your posture.

Now, think about a squat. You lower the weight so your butt's below your knees. During the squat, you maintain your posture with a flat back and balance through your feet. Your upper body and core are engaged. Then you reverse the motion and stand without tipping over. It's a far more active motion that requires the muscles of your *whole* body.

The other cool part about these functional movements is that they can be done with minimal equipment. A few sets of dumbbells are all you need to get started. If you travel often, last week's basic un-weighted movements are awesome for travel workouts. And many hotel gyms have dumbbells, so level 1 is something you could easily do while on the road. Even a heavy backpack can be used in place of weights.

Progressive Overload

There's a reason why many people plateau once they start strength training: they forget to progressively overload their muscles. In simpler terms, they never increase the weights used. It's fine to start with your bodyweight for many movements, but once you get stronger, slowly and incrementally use more weight.

The human body is amazingly adaptive, and you actually get stronger when you recover from your training. Recall that when you stress muscle, it ends up with

micro-damage that the body repairs. The repaired tissue is stronger than the original tissue, like what happens to a broken bone once it heals.

The idea is to slowly ramp up the weights over time to avoid plateauing. In the Core 4 program, I've sequenced both levels with the kind of progression that'll keep building your strength and obtain results. Over time, the reps and sets will change, so be sure to look at each workout closely.

For level 1, dumbbell weights are prescribed for many exercises. Slowly increase the weight over time when appropriate. If you completed each set and it was too easy, try going a little heavier next time. Select a weight that's challenging but still allows you to use great form. It's *never* worth trying to lift a heavier weight if the quality of your movement suffers.

For level 2, how much weight you'll use is up to you. If something is too heavy, make an adjustment. In other words, don't blindly follow the planned reps, sets, and loads if you aren't able to move well.

Day 8 Challenge: Work Out

Note that levels 1 and 2 are now on different plans going forward. Pick your favorite movements from last week for a dynamic warm-up. Complete all sets and reps of each movement before moving on to the next.

Make sure to track your sleep today.

LEVEL 1

GOBLET SQUATS—*4 sets of 10 reps*

Stand with your feet slightly wider than hip width, and hold a dumbbell or kettlebell in front of your chest. Inhale and engage your core as you hinge from your hips and bend your knees to lower your butt toward the floor, keeping your feet in a comfortable squat stance with your thighs a little lower than parallel. Exhale as you return to the starting position.

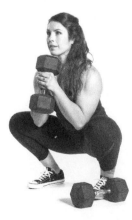

ALTERNATING LUNGES—*3 sets of 8 reps with each leg*

Stand with your feet under your hips, holding dumbbells in both hands. Step forward and bend your right knee to make a 90-degree angle with your right leg as you lower your left knee toward the floor. Drive through your front foot. Step forward with your left leg to bring your feet together. Repeat the movements on the opposite leg.

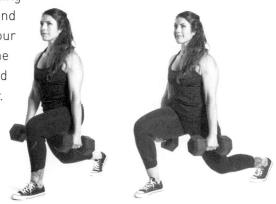

Pro Tips

» Make your step short enough that you can return to standing without swinging your torso.

» *To make it harder*, make them walking lunges, or hold the dumbbells over your head while you lunge.

PUSH-UPS—*3 sets of 8 reps*

Lie facedown on the floor and place your hands on the floor next to your body at about chest level, with your elbows close to your sides. Your body should look like an arrow if you could view it from above, not the letter T. Push your body up so that you're on your hands and toes, keeping your body in a straight line. Don't stick your butt up into the air or drop your butt too low. Bend your elbows to lower your chest toward the floor, and then push back up. As you push up, take a breath and keep your butt and core tight.

Pro Tip

» *To make it harder*, add weight on your back, or try clapping push-ups.

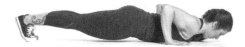

WAITER WALKS—*3 sets of 50 feet with each arm*

Stand with your feet under your hips and hold light- to moderate-weight dumbbells in each hand. Press your right dumbbell up toward the ceiling, actively pushing through your shoulder and keeping your right arm close to your head. Then walk with the dumbbell overhead. Pull your ribs down instead of flaring them out. Repeat the movements with your left arm.

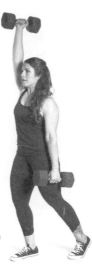

SEATED SIDE TWISTS—*3 sets of 8 reps on each side*

Sit on the floor with your knees bent, your feet flat on the floor, and a dumbbell held in both hands at chest height. Lean back, bringing your feet off the floor, and slowly twist your body to the right as you move the dumbbell toward your right hip. Keep your sit bones on the floor. Then rotate your body slowly to the left, moving the dumbbell toward your left hip. Keep the weight close to your body as you rotate from side to side.

SUPER(WO)MANS OR BIRD DOGS—*3 sets of 12 reps*

Lie facedown on the floor and extend your arms out in front of you. Inhale and then exhale as you engage your core and lift your arms and legs a few inches off the floor. Activate your back and butt muscles, moving slowly until you reach a comfortable maximum height. Hold for 1 to 3 seconds, then return to the starting position.

Pro Tips

» *To make it harder,* increase the reps.

» *To make it easier,* decrease the reps, or 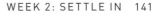 don't lift as far off the floor. You can also substitute with bird dogs: position yourself on all fours on the floor and extend one arm out in front of you while also extending the opposite leg out behind you, keeping your weight centered; then switch the arm and leg.

LEVEL 2

Starting this week, in level 2 you'll begin incorporating barbell lifts for the rest of the program. In order to make it simple, you'll use a system called *Rate of Perceived Exertion (RPE)* to guide your squats, deadlifts, presses, and power cleans. RPE is a scale to subjectively measure how hard you feel your body is working. You rate an exertion from 1 to 10 in difficulty, allowing you to tune in to how you're feeling on any one day and determine your level of effort.

There are several different RPE charts, but this is the one I recommend:

RPE Scale

1 Very, very light—the movement takes almost no effort

2 Light

3 Light—you can do several reps without a problem

4 Light to moderate

5 Moderate—a weight that gets your blood moving; a 50 percent effort

6 Moderate

7 Moderately heavy—it's getting challenging; you can do probably 5 to 7 reps

8 Heavy—you can do probably 2 to 4 reps with good form

9 Very heavy—not quite your maximum effort, but very hard; you can do probably 1 or 2 reps

10 Maximum effort—all-out exertion; you can do a single rep

Keep in mind that even though each workout lists the working sets for the barbell lifts, it's important to work up to these by including *warm-up sets*. In other words, don't just walk up to a barbell without warming up and try to do a set of squats at RPE 8! Including some warm-up sets helps your body get accustomed to the moves and adjust little by little to more challenging weights. I recommend starting with an empty bar and doing a set of 5 to 10 reps. Then try to give yourself at least 3 warm-up

sets of 5 reps before tucking into your working sets. If it's a higher RPE, maybe warm up a little more.

Let's go through an example of a squat workout. This is the first on your list of movements for today, so go ahead and give it a try.

BARBELL BACK SQUATS—*5 sets of 5 reps at RPE 5 (this RPE means you should feel a "moderate" effort—the weight should get your blood moving)*

Stand with a barbell resting across the meaty back of your shoulders, called the trapezius muscles, and held in an overhand grip. Don't let the barbell rest on your neck bones. Inhale, engage your core, squeeze your glutes, and hinge at the hip before bending your knees to lower your butt toward the floor until your thighs are parallel to the floor or slightly lower. Keep your neck neutral and your chest high, then return to the starting position, exhaling on the way up.

» **WARM-UP SET 1:** Squat the empty bar for 1 set of 10 reps. Rest 1 to 2 minutes or as needed.

» **WARM-UP SET 2:** Squat 1 set of 5 reps at RPE 3. Rest 1 to 2 minutes or as needed.

» **WARM-UP SET 3:** Squat 1 set of 5 reps at RPE 4. Rest 1 to 2 minutes or as needed.

» **WORKING SETS:** Squat 5 sets of 5 reps at RPE 5. Rest 2 to 4 minutes between sets or as needed.

Record in a journal the weights you used for all sets so you know where to start the next time you do these barbell back squats, and do the same for all the other barbell workouts.

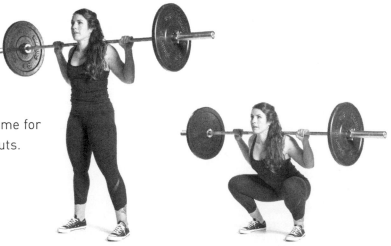

BARBELL SHOULDER PRESSES—*3 sets of 5 reps at RPE 5*

Stand with your feet under your hips and holding a barbell across the front of your shoulders with an overhand grip. Your hands should be slightly wider than shoulder width apart. Engage your core and press the barbell toward the ceiling. Maintain a neutral posture and pull your ribs down instead of flaring them out. Return to the starting position.

PULL-UPS—*4 sets of 5 reps*

Stand under a pull-up bar with your hands gripping the bar underhand or overhand (your choice) and shoulder width apart. Your thumbs should be wrapped all the way around the bar. Inhale as you engage your core and pull your body up until your chin clears the bar. Keep your neck neutral—don't crane your chin over the bar. Then lower back to the starting position with control to protect your shoulders.

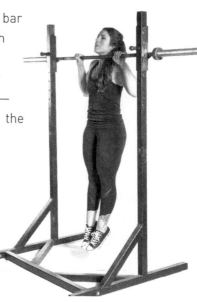

Pro Tips

» *To make it easier,* secure a band around the bar and place your feet in it to reduce the amount of weight you're pulling up. Or start at the top of the pull-up position and then lower yourself down instead of doing the complete rep.

SUPER(WO)MANS OR BIRD DOGS—*3 sets of 12 reps*

Lie facedown on the floor and extend your arms out in front of you. Engage your core and lift your arms and legs a few inches off the floor. Activate your back and butt muscles, moving slowly until you reach a comfortable maximum height. Hold for 1 to 3 seconds, then return to the starting position.

Pro Tips

» *To make it harder,* increase the reps.

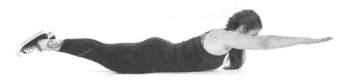

» *To make it easier,* decrease the reps, or don't lift as far off the floor. You can also substitute with bird dogs: position yourself on all fours on the floor and extend one arm out in front of you while also extending the opposite leg out behind you, keeping your weight centered; then switch the arm and leg.

DAY 9: THOUGHT AWARENESS

Part of strength training is learning how to focus your mind on what you're doing. When you "put your mind into your muscle," you'll see far more results from your workouts. Today's challenge asks you to peek in on what's happening in your mind from moment to moment. The purpose is to simply develop awareness of your thinking, when your mind is serving you and when it's not.

You really can't ever stop your thoughts. Sometimes they seep in like rain leaking through roof shingles . . . and sometimes they're as subtle as a torrential downpour. But instead of trying to stop thoughts, some of us keep harboring the same, and sometimes painful, thoughts.

We all tend to treat our thoughts as true, especially the painful ones. And often we act on our thoughts, which makes them feel even more real. Whether we're thinking about ourselves or about something someone did or said to us, our thoughts can be a source of much anxiety, fear, and sadness, especially when we play them over and over in our minds.

Your job today is not to stop your thoughts but to simply observe them objectively. Once you observe your thoughts, consider:

What's really going to serve you?

What's accurate regarding the situation?

Are you going to act on someone else's opinion or stay grounded in your truth?

Acting as an outside observer to your thoughts is a habit, and the good news is that it can be strengthened through practice.

Storytelling

How has human language been transmitted through the years? It all started with oral tradition, so it's no surprise that we're very good storytellers.

Yet our memories aren't as good as we think they are. When the brain processes and stores memories, it often alters the information. And studies have shown it's possible to introduce memories of events that didn't actually happen.

What this means is that when you replay a memory from your past, you may not be remembering it 100 percent accurately. Bad memories can make you relive your past in the present as well—a so-called self-fulfilling prophecy.

This may all sound a little disconcerting, but I think it's great news. It means the brain is adaptable, and we can keep learning new things for our entire lives.

The Power of Now

So what's the takeaway? Is it time to get upset and self-judgmental because of the stories you keep telling yourself or the thinking that drags you down? Hellllllllll no. The solution is to be aware without judging yourself and to stay grounded in the present.

Here's an example. When I was growing up, my stepdad once called me "the chubby one." Every time I thought of this memory, it hurt. It made me sad, and I created a narrative around it called "I'm Not Good Enough." For many, many years I lived and acted like it was true. Only in the last decade or so have I been able to see the story for what it is. It's something that happened to me thirty years ago, *but it's not happening to me right now*. Right now, I'm sitting in my lovely, safe home having just eaten lunch, typing away on my computer, and actually feeling quite content.

That's one way to stop your story mode from playing out in the present. I'm not saying to deny everything that's ever happened to you, nor that your experiences don't shape your worldview. But what I'm challenging you to do, when you get upset, anxious, or stressed out, is ask yourself this: "What is actually happening to me *right now*?"

My strategy for stopping the downward spiral into uncontrollable negative thinking is simple but effective. You'll remember it from the Pillar 3 chapter. It is called Stop, Breathe, and Do.

> **STOP.** Actually get a grip on where you are and what you're doing. Chances are you are safe and aren't experiencing any real threat. If you need to, sit and speak out loud or jot down where you are. For example, "Right now, I'm sitting in my lovely, safe home having just eaten lunch, typing away on my computer, and actually feeling quite content."
>
> **BREATHE.** Immediately start breathing deeply from your belly, not shallowly from your chest. Shallow breathing activates the fight-or-flight part of your nervous system. Breathe with a soft belly, taking slow, deep inhalations and even slower exhalations for one to two minutes.
>
> **DO.** Interrupt the thinking by picking up something that requires your focus. I've seen this work well when clients do something creative like knit or crochet, draw or doodle, chop veggies, play a musical instrument, garden, etc.

Day 9 Challenge: Track Your Story Mode

On a piece of scrap paper or in your phone, keep note of how many times your thoughts slip away from you. As a bonus, practice the three-step technique just mentioned: stop, breathe, and do.

Make sure to track your sleep today.

DAY 10: STRONG ARMS

Take a look at Day 9's challenge. Were you surprised at how often your thoughts take you away from the present? Keep practicing the stop, breathe, and do strategy as often as necessary to give the finger to your intrusive, negative, and self-defeating

thoughts—it works! Today, though, we'll focus on the body again—specifically your arms.

Having strong arms doesn't just mean you can open pickle jars by yourself . . . though that's a nice side benefit. Being strong enough to push and pull your body-weight—or more—is a fundamental expression of your body's potential.

In a practical sense, there are lots of reasons why having strong arms matters. Think of your daily routine. How often do you pick things up or put them away? If you play a sport, you likely use your arms quite a bit. That makes sense.

But here's where things take a serious tone. Even though, as women, our muscles are smaller, we have the same capacity to get stronger that men have. We're not bound to a lifetime of weakness simply because we aren't guys. Many of my clients say they want to get strong enough to do their first pull-up, and then they invariably take on a defeated tone before they even start: "But, Steph, I'll never get there. I'm just not strong."

Hogwash. Remember, your body has incredible potential for strength. However, our modern lifestyle allows us to hardly use our strength unless we actively choose to. So we lose it—at least for a little while.

What's really cool is that even though your strength might be lower right now, with consistency and training in functional movements, you'll build the capacity, stability, and power to do a pull-up. You might not get there in a month or two or even six, but with practice, you'll get there eventually. It's not a pipe dream. It's not a "Well, I'll never be able to." Strong arms are an expression of your innate human strength and capacity.

Healthy Shoulders

The shoulder is an incredibly complex joint with numerous muscular attachments that all play together nicely to create a glorious range of motion. However, when our muscles get bound up and full of knots, our range of motion becomes limited.

Let's focus on internal and external shoulder rotation. Internal rotation in a lift is a common flaw and one of the reasons you may struggle with overhead movements. If the shoulders internally rotate, causing the chest to dip or cave, it's common for the weight to drift forward. This position is very unstable. With lighter weights you may

How to Mobilize Your Shoulders

I want to point out a couple of my favorite mobility moves for pressing. Getting into better positions by mobilizing will allow you to achieve better range of motion. Remember to select at least some mobility drills related to the movements you're performing in a workout to get the most bang for your buck.

Here are two ways to prep for shoulder exercises:

Trap Softener

Place an empty barbell in a squat rack and add 10-pound plates on both ends. Secure the weights with clips. Move under the bar and stand at one end facing one plate. Lift that end of the bar and rest it on the meaty part of your trapezius muscle. Then move your arm from your side to overhead in one smooth movement. Do that 10 times on each side of your traps.

Lat Release

Lie on the floor on your back. Put a foam roller under your upper spine. Now roll slightly so your lat "meat" is on top of the roller—that's the latissimus dorsi muscle, which stretches across the mid-back up toward the shoulder. Go gently at first and roll up and down your lat 10 times. Repeat the movement on the other lat. You can adjust the pressure by raising or lowering your hips through the movement.

be able to get away with it (not that you should try to), but when things get heavy, it'll all fall apart.

When externally rotated, the joint is in a much more stable, safe position for supporting a load overhead. Stretch your right hand over your head with your palm up. Now act like you're screwing in a light bulb. That's external rotation. Feel it?!

Start getting aware of external rotation, especially when you're warming up and mobilizing. Practice with a PVC pipe, broomstick, or empty training bar to get the feel of external rotation. Develop an awareness when you're doing overhead work, and correct yourself when needed.

The ultimate goal is full range of motion. Missing internal rotation as part of your range of motion isn't good either!

Day 10 Challenge: Work Out

Again, movements from Week 1 make a dynamic warm-up. Complete all sets and reps of each movement before moving on to the next.

Make sure to track your sleep today.

LEVEL 1

SUITCASE DEADLIFTS—*4 sets of 10 reps*

Position your feet hip width apart and hold dumbbells or kettlebells next to your feet. Engage your core, squeeze your glutes, and come to a standing position by trying to push the floor away with your legs instead of lifting with your back. Keep your spine aligned throughout the movement, and keep the weights close to your body. Then hinge forward at the hip and return to the starting position. Be sure to keep your toes from lifting off the floor throughout the movement.

Pro Tip

» *To make it harder,* use a barbell.

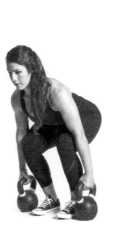

SPLIT SQUATS—*3 sets of 8 reps with each leg*

Stand with your feet under your hips and with dumbbells held at shoulder height. Step forward with your left leg into a lunge stance. Engage your core and gently lower your right knee toward the floor until both legs form 90-degree angles. Return to a standing position, then lower your right knee again. Do all reps on this leg before driving through your front foot, engaging your glutes and returning to the starting position. Repeat with opposite leg positions.

Pro Tip

» *To make it harder,* place your back foot up on a bench (to do a Bulgarian split squat).

ALTERNATING DUMBBELL ROWS—*3 sets of 8 reps*

Holding a dumbbell in your left hand, to begin with, stand with your right foot forward in a partial lunge and your body from your left heel to the top of your head forming almost a straight line. Keep your core engaged, your spine aligned, and your elbow close to your body as you pull the dumbbell up to your ribs, then lower it. You can rest your other hand on your knee or your leg for support. Repeat the movements on the opposite side.

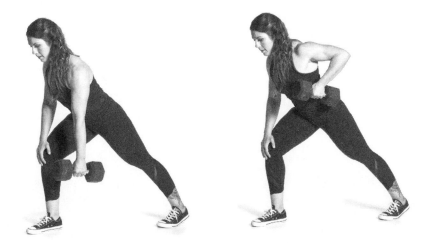

ALTERNATING DUMBBELL SHOULDER PRESSES—*3 sets of 8 reps with each arm*

Stand with your feet under your hips and with dumbbells in both hands held at shoulder height, with your knuckles facing your shoulders. Engage your core, squeeze your butt, and keep your neck neutral as you actively push up through the shoulder to raise one dumbbell toward the ceiling. Keep your arm close to your head. Also, pull your ribs down instead of flaring them out. Lower the dumbbell and repeat the movements with the opposite arm.

Pro Tip

» *To make it harder,* press both dumbbells up at the same time or use a barbell.

PLANKS—*4 sets of 20 seconds*

Lie on the floor facedown with your hands next to your chest and your elbows close to your sides. Take a breath and push your body up onto your toes and hands, engaging your core and keeping your body in a straight line. Don't stick your butt up in the air or let your hips sag. Hold this position, breathing normally.

Pro Tip

» *To make it harder,* add weight to your back, or lift one leg off the floor.

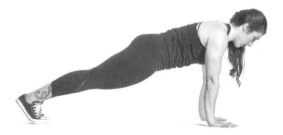

LEVEL 2

BARBELL DEADLIFTS—*1 set of 5 reps at RPE 5*

Stand with your feet under your hips with a barbell on the floor close to your shins. Hinge at the hips and grasp the barbell overhand with your hands positioned just outside your hips. Inhale, engage your core, squeeze your glutes, and push the floor away with your legs instead of lifting your back to raise the barbell. Keep your neck neutral and the barbell close to your body as you come to a standing position, exhaling on the way up. Be sure to keep your toes from lifting off the floor throughout the movement. Hinge forward at the hips, lower the weight to the floor, and return to the starting position.

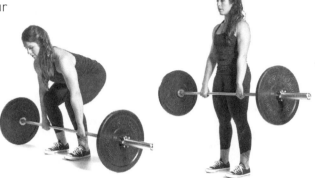

BARBELL POWER CLEANS—*3 sets of 4 reps at RPE 5*

Stand with your feet slightly wider than hip width apart and with a barbell on the floor in front of your feet. Hinge at the hips and grab the barbell overhand with your hands positioned just outside your hips. Lift it to your thighs, then push with your legs and jump as you bend your elbows to flip the bar up and shrug it to your shoulders. The power comes from your legs driving the bar up rather than pulling it with your arms. Stand in a partial squat with your knees slightly bent. Pause briefly, then return the bar to the floor.

Pro Tip

» *To make it harder,* use an unbalanced object like a sandbag, or receive the weight in a full squat clean.

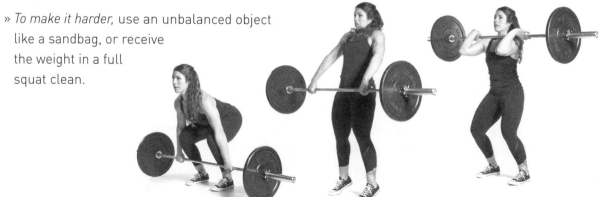

PUSH-UPS—*4 sets of 5 reps*

Lie facedown on the floor and place your hands on the floor next to your body at about chest level, with your elbows close to your sides. Your body should look like an arrow if you could view it from above, not the letter T. Push your body up so that you're on your hands and toes, keeping your body in a straight line. Don't stick your butt up into the air or drop your butt too low. Bend your elbows to lower your chest toward the floor, and then push back up. As you push up, take a breath and keep your butt and core tight.

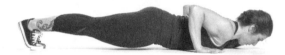

Pro Tip

» *To make it harder,* add weight on your back, or try clapping push-ups.

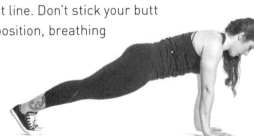

PLANKS—*4 sets of 20 seconds*

Lie on the floor facedown with your hands next to your chest and your elbows close to your sides. Take a breath and push your body up onto your toes and hands, engaging your core and keeping your body in a straight line. Don't stick your butt up in the air or let your hips sag. Hold this position, breathing normally.

Pro Tip

» *To make it harder,* add weight to your back, or lift one leg off the floor.

DAY 11: STAY HYDRATED

As you progress through the program, you should expect some ups and downs. Some days you may be rarin' to get after it in the gym. Other days . . . well, not so much. Do your best and shake off any guilt about a so-so workout. In other words, let it go!

We spend an awful lot of time talking about what we should eat, but what about drinking? (Not alcohol—#sorrynotsorry.) I'm talking about the concept of hydration in general.

Now, there are different approaches here. Some people hydrate like crazy, carrying around their plastic jugs like purses. You know who they are. (Maybe it's you!)

On the other hand, some people hardly ever drink. They're like human camels.

I'm not a huge fan of prescribing how much people should drink, but let's just say that too much is just as bad as not enough. When it comes down to it, your body automatically knows how to regulate your fluids. Drink enough that your blood volume increases and your kidneys start excreting more fluid. Your pee should be light in color—about the color of straw. If it's clear, you may be drinking too much. (If it's very dark, not enough.)

Common complaints related to dehydration include fatigue, headaches, cravings, irritability, and muscle cramps. The next time you feel tired in the middle of the day and reach for a coffee or sugar pick-me-up, make sure you're well hydrated.

Keeping Electrolytes in Balance

Electrolytes are the dissolved substances in cells that control a whole host of things, from nerve impulses to muscle contractions to regulating what goes across cell membranes. (See? They matter a whole lot.)

Let's get science-y again for a minute. You've heard of sodium, potassium, calcium, magnesium, and chloride. They're a few of the important electrolytes that must be delicately balanced to make sure you're a properly functioning hunk of muscle and bone.

If you drink too much—like really, really try to force it—it's possible to dilute your electrolyte levels so fast that your kidneys can't keep up. This isn't just undesirable; it can be fatal in extreme situations. This sometimes happens when it's very hot and electrolytes are being sweated out faster than they can be replenished, coupled with overdrinking water.

If you're an endurance athlete or you'll be outside for a long time and sweating a lot, use electrolyte tablets or drops that dissolve in water. Salt tablets are another option in extremely hot weather, but an ideal electrolyte additive will contain other electrolytes—like potassium and calcium—as well.

So how much should you drink? A good rule of thumb is half your bodyweight (measured in pounds) in ounces per day, but your actual needs vary with the climate, altitude, any medications you're taking, and your personal body chemistry.

Day 11 Challenge: Tune In to Your Hydration

To get a rough estimate of how hydrated you are, keep track of how much fluid you drink today, the color of your urine each time you pee, and the way you feel in relation to how much water you're drinking.

DAY 12: JANKY BITS

Janky bits are what I call those parts of your body that aren't quite functioning at 100 percent. You know the ones I'm talking about—the pieces that limit your mobility, feel stiff or achy, or otherwise interfere with feeling flexible, strong, and stable.

Mobility isn't something that "just gets better." If you ignore them, these jank-a-riffic parts don't improve.

You may *know* you need to work on your mobility, but unless you devote some time to it, you're not going to magically fix your overhead position or be able to get low enough for a deep squat. You need to keep your tissues from getting bound up.

That means enabling your muscles and tissues to slide over each other properly; preventing your connective tissue from getting gunky or stiff; and all manner of reducing inflammation thanks to diet, sleep, and recovery practices.

You don't need to spend hours every day doing mobility work, but just a few minutes before and after your workout can help a *lot*. The key is to pick a couple of mobility drills that hit the body parts you'll be working on any given day. That might mean doing work on your ankles and hips before you squat or loosening up your shoulders when you're going to do presses. Work smarter, not harder.

Tools of the Trade

Are you über stiff? Do you have unicorn-level special mobility issues? If you're just getting started, I recommend these tools:

- foam roller
- lacrosse ball

These are a simple way to address mobility—and they can help save you the cost and pain of chronic injuries that may come from training with a limited range of motion.

What's that saying? "An ounce of prevention is worth a pound of cure."

Day 12 Challenge: Work Out

Movements from last week make a great dynamic warm-up. Complete all sets and reps of each movement before moving on to the next.

LEVEL 1

GLUTE BRIDGES—*3 sets of 12 reps*

Lie on your back with your knees bent, your feet flat on the floor and close to your hips, and your arms at your sides on the floor. Engage your core and squeeze your butt as you slowly drive your hips up toward the ceiling so that your body is in a straight line from head to knees. Keep your knees parallel to each other; don't let them collapse in or out. Slowly lower your hips back to the starting position.

Pro Tip

» *To make it harder,* lift up one leg at a time from the bridge position.

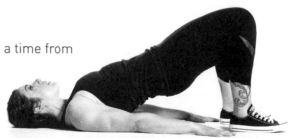

SINGLE-LEG DEADLIFTS—*3 sets of 6 reps with each leg*

Stand with your feet hip width apart and with dumbbells in both hands. Engage your core and keep your spine aligned as you shift your weight onto your left foot. Hinge forward at the hip to lower the weights until they reach the middle of your left shin as you extend your right leg behind you, balancing on your left. Feel your glute and hamstring on the standing leg activate, and soften the standing knee—don't lock it. Keep your hips square. Rise back to the standing position and do all the reps before switching legs and repeating the movements.

Pro Tip

» *To make it easier,* do this move without dumbbells and put one hand on a wall to keep your balance.

PULL-UPS—*4 sets of 4 to 6 reps*

Stand under a pull-up bar with your hands gripping the bar underhand or overhand (your choice) and shoulder width apart. Your thumbs should be wrapped all the way around the bar. Inhale as you engage your core and pull your body up until your chin clears the bar. Keep your neck neutral—don't crane your chin over the bar. Then lower back to the starting position with control to protect your shoulders.

Pro Tips

» *To make it easier,* secure a band around the bar and place your feet in it to reduce the amount of weight you're pulling up. Or start at the top of the pull-up position and then lower yourself down instead of doing the complete rep.

MOUNTAIN CLIMBERS—*3 sets of 10 reps with each leg*

Get on the floor in the plank position, with your hands shoulder width apart. Engage your core as you quickly pull one knee toward your chest, just touching your foot to the floor before extending that leg back again. Repeat the movement with the opposite leg. Continue to alternate legs.

Pro Tip

» *To make it harder,* increase the pace.

HOLLOW ROCKS—*4 sets of 10 reps*

Lie on your back with your arms extended above your head. Engage your core and raise your legs and arms at the same time, pointing your toes and keeping your arms close to your ears. Press your lower back to the floor as you rock lightly back and forth, maintaining the same body position and breathing normally. Relax down into your starting position.

Pro Tip

» *To make it harder,* hang by your arms from a pull-up bar instead, squeeze your butt, brace your core, and pull your knees up toward your elbows, crunching your abs.

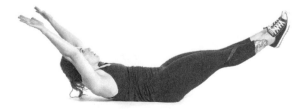

LEVEL 2

BARBELL BACK SQUATS—*5 sets of 5 reps at RPE 6*

Stand with a barbell resting across the meaty back of your shoulders, called the trapezius muscles, and held in an overhand grip. Don't let the barbell rest on your neck bones. Inhale, engage your core, squeeze your glutes, and hinge at the hip before bending your knees to lower your butt toward the floor until your thighs are parallel to the floor or slightly lower. Keep your neck neutral and your chest high, then return to the starting position, exhaling on the way up.

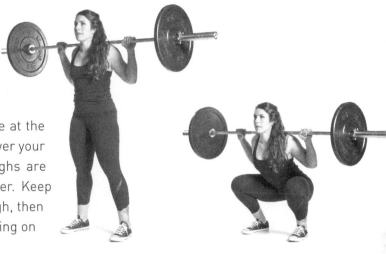

BARBELL SHOULDER PRESSES—*3 sets of 4 reps at RPE 6*

Stand with your feet under your hips and holding a barbell across the front of your shoulders with an overhand grip. Your hands should be slightly wider than shoulder width apart. Engage your core and press the barbell toward the ceiling. Maintain a neutral posture and pull your ribs down instead of flaring them out. Return to the starting position.

PULL-UPS—*4 sets of 5 reps*

Stand under a pull-up bar with your hands gripping the bar underhand or overhand (your choice) and shoulder width apart. Your thumbs should be wrapped all the way around the bar. Inhale as you engage your core and pull your body up until your chin clears the bar. Keep your neck neutral— don't crane your chin over the bar. Then lower back to the starting position with control to protect your shoulders.

Pro Tips

» *To make it easier,* secure a band around the bar and place your feet in it to reduce the amount of weight you're pulling up. Or start at the top of the pull-up position and then lower yourself down instead of doing the complete rep.

HOLLOW ROCKS—*4 sets of 10 reps*

Lie on your back with your arms extended above your head. Engage your core and raise your legs and arms at the same time, pointing your toes and keeping your arms close to your ears. Press your lower back to the floor as you rock lightly back and forth, maintaining the same body position and breathing normally. Relax down into your starting position.

Pro Tip

» *To make it harder,* hang by your arms from a pull-up bar instead, squeeze your butt, brace your core, and pull your knees up toward your elbows, crunching your abs.

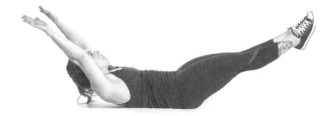

DAY 13: BREATHE AND RELAX

Fitness programs often focus on exercise with little attention paid to rest and recovery. Yet it's during recovery days like today that your body rebuilds itself and gets stronger. That's just one reason relaxation is critical to becoming more resilient.

You live in a constantly connected world. Between work and personal life, you're likely interacting with people most of the day. You get sucked into dramas unfolding around you—either consciously or unconsciously—and you probably don't unplug unless you're asleep.

Resilience is crucial for your mind as much as your body. In this modern age, you've got stress from relationships, money, work, and your own expectations of what you "should" be doing. It's enough to make you sick. Literally.

Some amount of stress is good. When you train, you're physically stressed. Stressed muscles repair and rebuild stronger than before. When you tweak your diet, that can cause stress too, both physical and psychological. But the key is how much stress you're under and whether you're recovering from it. Shit happens in life, and it's not uncommon to have multiple stressful events slam you at once. When stress is chronic and you don't give yourself enough recovery, you get weaker.

Taking Time Out

Some people are more resilient than others, but nobody is completely immune to stress. While you can't avoid every situation that could cause stress, you can actively work to reduce it.

Sometimes it's as simple as shifting how you approach things. You might change your fitness routine to something less intense. Or take better care of yourself through the food you nourish your body with. Or take time out, even for five minutes, to quiet your body and mind. (And, no, sleeping doesn't count.)

Try to sit or lie quietly with your eyes closed and focus on your breathing, or think of a particular word or phrase. "Sit spots" are great: sit for ten minutes and observe the world around you and how your body feels. You don't have to do hours of meditation.

Staying still for five minutes without distractions, like a phone or computer, might be hard at first. The app Headspace provides a great start. Or check out *Meditation Minis,* a podcast-based meditation tool created by my friend Chel Hamilton.

Incorporate a guided mediation three times a week to start. If you want to do more, fantastic. Eventually shoot for daily, up to twenty minutes at a time. If that weirds you out, start with five or ten minutes and slowly add to that.

Belly Breathing

The simplest intervention when you feel yourself getting stressed out is to breathe. As I mentioned earlier in the book, too often when we get stressed and slip into fight-or-flight mode (triggering the sympathetic nervous system), our breathing gets very shallow. Deep breathing through the belly works wonders to offset that and get the body to return to the rest-and-digest mode (tapping into the parasympathetic nervous system).

What's clutch is that you can do it anywhere under any circumstances. You don't need special equipment or a particular space. Just sit and breathe deeply, from your belly, not shallowly from your shoulders and chest. Start with three deep belly breaths. Do more if you want to.

Some people find the technique of box breathing—sometimes called four-square breathing—to be extremely helpful. It's simple:

Stand, sit, or lie down comfortably.

Breathe in through your nose, focusing on expanding your belly, for a count of four.

Hold for a count of four.

Slowly exhale through a slightly open mouth for a count of four.

Hold for a count of four.

Repeat as needed, up to a couple of minutes.

You may find the breath-holding to be a bit intense at first. If that's the case, simply do the inhale and the exhale for a four count. This is also a great technique for getting back to sleep in the middle of the night. For maximum parasympathetic activation, exhale for twice as long as you inhale: four in and eight out.

Day 13 Challenge: Complete a Guided Meditation

Follow a guided meditation of five, ten, or twenty minutes. A five- or ten-minute meditation can be done anywhere; you may want to be at home for a twenty-minute one.

For a seated meditation, choose a comfortable sitting position. That could be in a chair with your feet flat on the floor. Or, if your feet don't comfortably sit flat on the floor, put a folded-up blanket underneath your feet to elevate them.

You can also sit on the floor. You may want to use a folded blanket to support your sit bones. Do whatever is most comfortable for you. For a reclining meditation, you may want to lie on a yoga mat or a blanket on the floor.

OPTIONAL WEEKEND WORKOUT. Do the following exercises, one after another, starting a new one each minute. Use a clock or timer to keep track of the minutes. Start the sequence with eight hollow rocks, then rest for the remainder of the first minute. At the start of the next minute, do ten mountain climbers, then rest for the remainder of that minute. At the start of the next minute, do twelve bodyweight squats, then rest for the remainder of that minute. Complete the sequence four times, for a total of 12 minutes.

HOLLOW ROCKS—*8 reps*

Lie on your back with your arms extended above your head. Engage your core and raise your legs and arms at the same time, pointing your toes and keeping your arms close to your ears. Press your lower back to the floor as you rock lightly back and forth, maintaining the same body position and breathing normally. Relax down into your starting position.

Pro Tip

» *To make it harder,* hang by your arms from a pull-up bar instead, squeeze your butt, brace your core, and pull your knees up toward your elbows, crunching your abs.

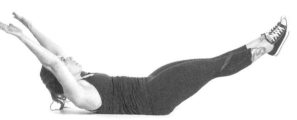

MOUNTAIN CLIMBERS—*5 reps per leg*

Get on the floor in the plank position, with your hands shoulder width apart. Engage your core as you quickly pull one knee toward your chest, just touching your foot to the floor before extending that leg back again. Repeat the movement with the opposite leg. Continue to alternate legs.

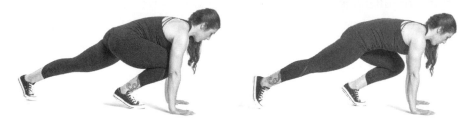

SQUATS—*12 reps*

Stand with your feet under your hips. Keeping your feet flat on the floor, engage your core as you push your hips back and bend your knees, lowering until your thighs are a little lower than parallel to the floor (or as low as feels comfortable). Go as low as you can while keeping a neutral spine. Your knees should track over your feet, and your chest should remain up. Then return to the starting position.

DAY 14: EMPTY BATTERY

You're two weeks into the Core 4 program. How does your body feel? With six work-outs under your belt, you may already notice a difference, especially when it comes to feeling more like a badass. And the more workouts you do, the more you'll own that. But for today's challenge, I want you to slow down a bit.

When you think of your energy, your thoughts might automatically drift to topics like sleep or recovery practices. You might even think that recharging your energy takes many hours or involves difficult tasks.

Sure, you need to actively recharge, but you can also take steps to decrease the constant and severe drain of your energies. Human beings aren't robots. Your energy naturally fluctuates throughout the day, and you certainly aren't meant to work hard without taking breaks.

In the Pillar 4 chapter you learned about two types of rhythms in human biology: circadian and ultradian. The circadian rhythm is often called the internal clock and governs your daily cycles of sleeping and waking. The ultradian rhythm is shorter and occurs multiple times in a day. It controls things like energy level, appetite, hormone release, and body temperature.

All this is to say that since cycles are part of your biology, it makes good sense to renew your energy throughout your day.

Take frequent short breaks. Do something to recharge, whether it's active or passive. Checking email, surfing the internet, or getting lost in social media may keep you busy, but that won't top up your energy.

If you can't take a break frequently, make sure your breaks are high quality. Eat a meal. Take a walk. Meditate. Get in a short workout.

Energy Is Time

What's the number one energy complaint people have? It's also the number one reason given for not exercising: "I don't have time to take a break."

It may sound surprising, but, yes, when your energy is being taxed and you're in survival mode, time seems to slip away from you. Are you multitasking your butt off and ending up with a bunch of half-done projects? Maybe you're not as efficient as you think you are. Research suggests multitasking is less efficient than sticking with one task until it's complete and that switching rapidly back and forth between tasks drains energy. A simple thing you can do is set a timer for thirty minutes and work on a single task with minimal distraction.

Day 14 Challenge: Prep Meals for Next Week

See the beginning of the next chapter for the upcoming week's shopping list and what to prep.

Kitchen Hacks for Saving Time

Spending all day hovering over a stove probably isn't your idea of fun. Yet some people seem to have it mastered. What do they know that you don't?

They've developed systems and shortcuts to make food prep and cooking more efficient. These are the things that save me tons of time in the kitchen:

Use a slow cooker or Instant Pot.

Cook in bulk. Gonna roast a tray of veggies? Roast two. Slow cooking a chicken? Put two in there. Making your favorite one-skillet recipe? Double it. You'll have instant leftovers.

When preparing soups or stews, double the batch and freeze the extra for later. That way you'll always have food in the freezer if you're in a pinch.

After you come home from grocery shopping, immediately wash and organize your veggies. Or take the time to prep them for the next day's cook-up by chopping, peeling, and storing them for the next day.

Make veggie bags. Chop your fresh veggies, sprinkle in herbs and spices, and store the bags in the fridge for the days ahead. They're not going to lose nutrient content that fast. Plus, if having them prepped means you'll eat *them* instead of pizza, it's worth it. Just save the salt until you're ready to roast them because the veggies will get soggy.

Fresh herbs are great to have on hand, but unless you store them properly, they'll dry out in a flash or get soggy and moldy. Here's how to keep them fresh for up to a week: Rinse the herbs with water and gently shake them out. Wrap them in a paper towel, then slide them into a ziplock bag. Keep the bag unsealed and refrigerated. Alternatively, fill a small jar with water and place the stems of the herb in the water. Slide a ziplock bag over the top and refrigerate.

Always keep your pantry well stocked so you can reach in and grab something to make a quick meal at a moment's notice. My faves: crushed tomatoes, coconut milk, apple cider vinegar, and avocado or coconut oil.

Shop the sales and buy in bulk. I have one of those little vacuum sealers that I use to portion and freeze meat so it doesn't get freezer burn.

Keep it simple. Listen, nobody's got time to make a five-course dinner on a busy weeknight. Stick to the basics, and you can't go wrong.

WEEK 3

Hit Your Stride

Week 2 is in the books! I'm stoked for your progress. Remember, it's small, consistent changes that add up to big results over time, so stay with it. Last week you did your first workouts with weights—and learned why a strong body is key to health. Keep up the great work and try to do a little more this week. It's normal to get scared about adding weight, but here's where that mindfulness lesson comes in handy: Notice the difference between something that's challenging and maybe a little outside your comfort zone versus something that's unsafe. Your body will tell you. Last week you also examined why recharging your batteries is vital to your health, and you learned some indispensable breathing techniques to help introduce a sense of calm . . . at any time!

Straight up, Week 3 is where women commonly lose some steam. It's seems weird (or is it?) because you're *finally* getting into a groove. But that's exactly the point: we humans get bored so easily. We're constantly seeking novelty, and the two-week mark is when people often bail from plans, even if those plans are working. It's just that the dopamine buzz has worn off. Not you, my friend! This week, let your process goals and the power of your new tools carry you through. Now might also be the time to seek out an accountability buddy if you're sensing the spark wearing off.

Week 3 Shopping List

Bacon (8 ounces plus
    4 slices)
Cheddar cheese, shredded
    full-fat (2 ounces),
    optional
Chicken wings (2 pounds)
Eggs (16)
Italian pork sausage
    (1 pound)
Lamb chops (2 pounds)
Sirloin steak (1 pound)

Avocados (2)
Bananas (2)
Carrots (3)
Cherry tomatoes (1 pint)
Cilantro, fresh (1 bunch),
    optional
Cucumber (1)
Garlic (1 head)
Green cabbage (1)
Green leaf lettuce (1)
Jicama (1)
Kale (1 bunch)
Lemon (1)
Limes (4) + Lime (1), optional

Mint, fresh (1 bunch)
Parsley, fresh (1 bunch)
Rosemary, fresh (4 sprigs)
Sweet potatoes (3)
Spinach (2 8-ounce bags)
Summer squash (2 pounds)
Swiss chard (1 bunch)
Yellow onions (2)
Yukon gold potatoes
    (2 pounds)

Almond milk (1 cup)
Ancho chili powder
    (3 teaspoons)
Avocado oil mayonnaise
    (¼ cup)
Chia seeds (2 tablespoons)
Chicken broth, low sodium
    (6 cups)
Chipotle pepper, ground
    (¼ teaspoon)
Cinnamon, ground
    (2 teaspoons)
Coconut milk (1 tablespoon)
Coconut, shredded and
    unsweetened (1 cup)

Cumin, ground (½ teaspoon)
Duck fat (2 tablespoons)
Extra-virgin olive oil or ghee
Flaxseed, ground (½ cup)
Garlic powder (¾ teaspoon)
Harissa sauce, mild
    (2 tablespoons)
Hemp hearts
    (2 tablespoons)
Honey (2 tablespoons)
Medjool dates (2)
Onion powder
    (1½ teaspoons)
Oregano, dried (¼ teaspoon)
Parsley, dried (½ teaspoon)
Pasta, gluten-free (8 ounces
    uncooked)
Rosemary, dried
    (½ teaspoon)
Salt and pepper
Smoked paprika
    (1 teaspoon)
Thyme, dried (¼ teaspoon)
Vanilla extract (2 teaspoons)

DAY 14

For this day's breakfast, lunch, and dinner, eat leftovers from the previous week.

Meals to prep:

» Steak Cobb Salad with Southwestern Ranch Dressing (page 267), dressing stored on the side

» Garlic Lamb Chops with Herb Gremolata (page 278)

» Cabbage, Bacon, and Noodles (page 271)

» Banana Cinnamon No-Oatmeal (page 260)

Other prep:

» 3 sweet potatoes, roast

» 2 8-ounce bags spinach, steam

DAY 15

BREAKFAST: Banana Cinnamon No-Oatmeal + steamed spinach

LUNCH: Steak Cobb Salad with Southwestern Ranch Dressing + roasted sweet potato

DINNER: Garlic Lamb Chops with Herb Gremolata + Cabbage, Bacon, and Noodles

DAY 16

BREAKFAST: Savory Ham and Egg Cups + steamed spinach

LUNCH: Garlic Lamb Chops with Herb Gremolata + Cabbage, Bacon, and Noodles

DINNER: Steak Cobb Salad with Southwestern Ranch Dressing + roasted sweet potato

DAY 17

BREAKFAST: Banana Cinnamon No-Oatmeal + steamed spinach

LUNCH: Steak Cobb Salad with Southwestern Ranch Dressing + roasted sweet potato

DINNER: Garlic Lamb Chops with Herb Gremolata + Cabbage, Bacon, and Noodles

DAY 18

BREAKFAST: Banana Cinnamon No-Oatmeal + steamed spinach

LUNCH: Steak Cobb Salad with Southwestern Ranch Dressing

DINNER: Hearty Tuscan Kale Soup (prepare today)

Meals to prep:

» Honey Harissa Chicken Wings (page 281)

» Hearty Tuscan Kale Soup (page 264)

» Smoky Duck Fat Potato Wedges (page 275)

Other prep:

» 2 pounds summer squash, roast

» 6 eggs, hard-boil

» 1 bunch swiss chard, steam

DAY 19

BREAKFAST: Hard-boiled eggs + Smoky Duck Fat Potato Wedges + steamed swiss chard

LUNCH: Honey Harissa Chicken Wings + roasted summer squash

DINNER: Hearty Tuscan Kale Soup

DAY 20

BREAKFAST: Hard-boiled eggs + steamed swiss chard

LUNCH: Hearty Tuscan Kale Soup

DINNER: Honey Harissa Chicken Wings + Smoky Duck Fat Potato Wedges + roasted summer squash

DAY 15: RECOVERY

Yesterday's challenge taught you about the importance of taking frequent breaks—real breaks that reboot your system. Today you'll learn about the importance of recovery and how to build more of it into your day. When you're resting, you're simply not moving. It's passive. Lying on the couch equals resting. Taking a day off from working out equals resting.

Recovery is a whole other thing, and it's one way to recharge your energy pillar. It's an *active* process of things you can do to improve your body and help it restore from the wear and tear of daily life as well as exercise.

Recovery techniques renew your body and your mind. Examples include things like

Acupuncture

Active release technique, or ART

Chiropractic

Cold therapy, or cryotherapy

Contrast baths or showers

Epsom salt baths

Foam rolling

Massage

Meditation

Restorative yoga

Sauna

Stretching and mobility work

Very light cardio

On days when you don't exercise, try to do something for active recovery, even if it's for only five or ten minutes.

Avoid Overtraining

When strength training, the eccentric—lowering—component of a lift is especially taxing on muscle fibers. When you don't allow enough recovery time between workouts, you'll feel it. Your coordination tanks. Your endurance slides. Your mental game is off. These are all cues to notice.

In the beginning, these signs of overwork might not seem serious, but if you ignore these signs without proper recovery, you can set yourself up for some serious bother. When lackluster nutrition, physical stress from too much exercise—either amount or intensity—and poor recovery combine, you may wind up in a state called "overtrained."

Performance dips can be accompanied by hormonal imbalances, particularly within the hypothalamic-pituitary-adrenal (HPA) axis or the hypothalamic-pituitary-thyroid (HPT) axis. Without getting too technical, let's just say that messing with your cortisol levels and thyroid hormones is not good.

The insidious part is that the dip in performance from overtraining often causes a person to think their problems are a result of too *little* exercise, so they work out *more* and the cycle worsens.

So how do you know if you should take a day off from exercise? Check in with your body when you start your workout. If the weights feel heavier than they should or you feel sluggish and uncoordinated, that's a sign that you need more recovery time. It's normal to feel some minor muscle soreness and even some mental discomfort when you start strength training because you're stretching your comfort zone . . . and that's a good thing! But if your body is too achy or stiff (and that feeling doesn't go away when you warm up), you can't maintain good form, or you feel unstable, it's okay to change up what you're doing or lower the weights. And it's totally fine to quit a workout if your intuition is telling you, "Not today."

Maybe that means you swap your workout for a walk instead or you do some light stretching or you just go home and take a hot bath. The more you listen to your body's signals, the better you'll get at recognizing the difference between your brain throwing a fake hissy fit (which you can push through) and overtraining.

I always say "Live to lift another day." Skipping a session here or there or modifying the workout to honor your body doesn't mean you lose all of your gains. And some-

times an extra rest day is exactly what you need! Remember, you get stronger when you *recover from* your workouts.

The takeaway? Working out more won't always give you better results. Now you have more insight into why the program is designed with three strength days a week and not more!

Day 15 Challenge: Work Out

Note that movements from Week 2 make a dynamic warm-up. Complete all sets and reps of each movement before moving on to the next.

LEVEL 1

SPLIT SQUATS—*4 sets of 8 reps with each leg*

Stand with your feet under your hips and with dumbbells held at shoulder height. Step forward with your left leg into a lunge stance. Engage your core and gently lower your right knee toward the floor until both legs form 90-degree angles. Return to a standing position, then lower your right knee again. Do all reps on this leg before driving through your front foot, engaging your glutes, and returning to the starting position. Repeat with opposite leg positions.

Pro Tip

» *To make it harder,* place your back foot up on a bench (to do a Bulgarian split squat).

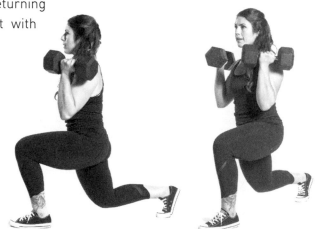

SUMO DEADLIFTS—*4 sets of 10 reps*

Stand with your feet about six to eight inches outside your hips and hold dumbbells or a kettlebell in front of your thighs with an overhand grip. Engage your core and keep your neck neutral as you hinge forward, bend your knees, and lower the weights until they touch the floor. Remember to push the floor away with your legs instead of lifting with your back. Return to the starting position, keeping the weights close to your body.

BENCH OR FLOOR PRESSES—*3 sets of 8 reps*

Lie on your back on a weight bench with your feet flat on the floor, or on the floor with your knees bent and your feet flat on the floor. Hold dumbbells in your hands next to your shoulders. Drive your feet into the floor and engage your core as you press the weights toward the ceiling and just outside your shoulder width. Bend your elbows and slowly lower the weights until they touch your shoulders, then press back up, focusing on your chest and triceps. Let your elbows touch the floor if you're on the floor.

Pro Tip

» *To make it harder,* do barbell bench presses.

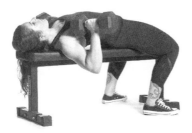
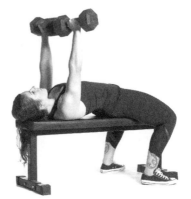

DIPS—*3 sets of 6 reps*

Sit on a sturdy bench or box with your hands next to you and your feet about twelve inches in front of your hips. Slide your bum off the bench, and keeping your body close to the bench, bend your arms to slowly lower your body a few inches below the bench, then drive back up, using your triceps, to the starting position.

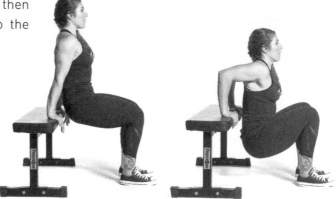

Pro Tips

» *To make it easier,* set your feet closer to your body.

» *To make it harder,* set your feet farther from your body.

PLANKS—*3 sets of 30 seconds*

Lie on the floor facedown with your hands next to your chest and your elbows close to your sides. Take a breath and push your body up onto your toes and hands, engaging your core and keeping your body in a straight line. Don't stick your butt up in the air or let your hips sag. Hold this position, breathing normally.

Pro Tip

» *To make it harder,* add weight to your back, or lift one leg off the floor.

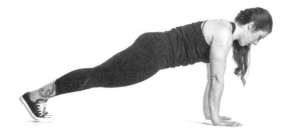

LEVEL 2

BARBELL BACK SQUATS—*5 sets of 5 reps at RPE 6*

Stand with a barbell resting across the meaty back of your shoulders, called the trapezius muscles, and held in an overhand grip. Don't let the barbell rest on your neck bones. Inhale, engage your core, squeeze your glutes, and hinge at the hip before bending your knees to lower your butt toward the floor until your thighs are parallel to the floor or slightly lower. Keep your neck neutral and your chest high, then return to the starting position, exhaling on the way up.

BARBELL POWER CLEANS—*3 sets of 3 reps at RPE 6*

Stand with your feet slightly wider than hip width apart and with a barbell on the floor in front of your feet. Hinge at the hips and grab the barbell overhand with your hands positioned just outside your hips. Lift it to your thighs, then push with your legs and jump as you bend your elbows to flip the bar up and shrug it to your shoulders. The power comes from your legs driving the bar up rather than pulling it with your arms. Stand in a partial squat with your knees slightly bent. Pause briefly, then return the bar to the floor.

Pro Tip

» *To make it harder,* use an unbalanced object like a sandbag, or receive the weight in a full squat clean.

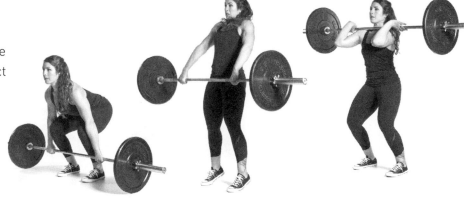

PUSH-UPS—*4 sets of 5 reps*

Lie facedown on the floor and place your hands on the floor next to your body at about chest level, with your elbows close to your sides. Your body should look like an arrow if you could view it from above, not the letter T. Push your body up so that you're on your hands and toes, keeping your body in a straight line. Don't stick your butt up into the air or drop your butt too low. Bend your elbows to lower your chest toward the floor, and then push back up. As you push up, take a breath and keep your butt and core tight.

Pro Tip

» *To make it harder,* add weight on your back, or try clapping push-ups.

SEATED SIDE TWISTS—*3 sets of 8 reps on each side*

Sit on the floor with your knees bent, your feet flat on the floor, and a dumbbell held in both hands at chest height. Lean back, bringing your feet off the floor, and slowly twist your body to the right as you move the dumbbell toward your right hip. Keep your sit bones on the floor. Then rotate your body slowly to the left, moving the dumbbell toward your left hip. Keep the weight close to your body as you rotate from side to side.

DAY 16: COOL THE FLAMES

Welcome to Day 16! You're past the halfway point of the Core 4 program, so give yourself a proverbial pat on the back. You got this! Today let's get out our mental microscopes and look inside the amazing organisms we too often take for granted. Understanding the different types of inflammation in your body can help you tell the difference between what's normal and what's not.

First, there are two main types of inflammation: acute and chronic. *Acute inflammation* is a good thing. For example, if you fall and twist your ankle, it starts to swell and gets red and hot. Another example is when your body is fighting an infection, such as the flu.

Blood flow increases to the area if the injury is localized, and depending on the infection or injury, the body may mount a larger-scale immune system response. (That's one of the reasons why your whole body aches if you get the flu.) Acute inflammation is part of the body's natural healing process. Think of it like a fast-burning fire. It may rage and flame up, but soon it's out.

On the other hand, we can have chronic, systemic inflammation. *Chronic inflammation* is a longer-term process, and "systemic" means it affects the whole system, or body. If acute inflammation is like a fast-burning fire, chronic is like smoldering ashes. It's there in the background, heating things up.

The causes of chronic, systemic inflammation may include:

- a damaged gut lining (increased intestinal permeability) that allows foreign particles into the bloodstream
- inflammatory foods, like sugar, alcohol, gluten, and some types of dairy
- insufficient sleep
- insulin resistance
- disrupted gut flora (dysbiosis)
- hormonal imbalances
- environmental toxins

When this type of inflammation goes unchecked, you may experience:

- fatigue
- body aches and injuries that don't heal well
- infections
- skin or gut issues
- allergies or food sensitivities
- autoimmune disorders

Studies continue to draw links between chronic inflammation and diseases such as diabetes, cardiovascular disease, and cancer.

How to Cool the Flames

Recognizing that inflammation—both acute and chronic—occurs is one thing; knowing how to reduce inflammation on a daily basis is where you want to take action. The good news is that many practices we've highlighted in this book reduce inflammation.

Let's start with food. The most anti-inflammatory foods are real, whole, unprocessed meats, eggs, veggies, fruits, and healthy fats and oils, like avocado, nuts, and seeds. Culinary spices like ginger and turmeric can also help reduce inflammation. However, if you suspect you have specific food sensitivities, I recommend doing a structured thirty-day elimination plan to gain more insight into your system.

The bottom line is that cheap processed junk food usually contains pro-inflammatory ingredients, like sugar and industrial vegetable oils. You can make a massive change in your inflammatory food intake by simply shifting away from processed foods. Substances like caffeine, alcohol, and other drugs can also ramp up inflammation, so consider cutting back if needed.

You can also support a healthy gut by consuming gut-boosting foods, such as bone broth and probiotic-rich fermented foods. And sleep and stress reduction cannot be overlooked; both a lack of sleep and a stressed-out daily life promote inflammation.

Day 16 Challenge: Revisit your Personal Pillar Plan

Take a few minutes to assess where you are. Have any pillars changed? If so, make adjustments to the actions you planned out. Remember, the plan is fluid and can change over time.

DAY 17: PRE- AND POST-WORKOUT EATS

Changing the way you eat is one of the easiest ways to reduce inflammation. It's simple: put crap food in your body daily and your body will feel like crap. The choices you make food-wise around your workouts can have a big impact on your performance—and the results afterward. The number one question I get from exercisers is "Do I need

to eat something before and after I work out?" If I had a dollar for every time this was asked, I'd be sipping frozen kombucha cocktails on a beach somewhere.

Pre-Workout Eats

Take a look at the Pre- and Post-Workout Cheat Sheet later in this section (page 185). Pre-workout, or preWO, refers to what you eat fifteen to sixty minutes prior to your workout. Whether you eat depends on a couple of things:

> Are you trying to actively gain mass? If yes, eat a preWO. You need to eat more often if you're on a program to gain lots of extra muscle.

> Did you eat within two or three hours of your workout? If yes, you may not feel hungry or want to eat again. That's fine.

Okay, so if you're not on a mass-gain program and you've eaten a meal less than two or three hours ago, you probably don't *need* a preWO. Your last meal is being digested and absorbed. Eating too much food too close to your workout means that it may sit in your stomach and leave you feeling bloated or nauseated.

If you ate properly the day before, your glycogen—that long chain of stored glucose—should be topped off in your muscle and ready to get you through your workout. If you do feel peckish or your stomach is rumbling because you're so hungry, eat a bit of protein and a bit of fat.

Why Protein?

The preWO's primary function is to jump-start recovery before a training session by providing the raw materials to repair muscle and to give you a bit of fat to take the edge off. You don't need a lot of carbohydrates because you want to teach your body to use what you've stored. And if you use *that* up, you want to teach it to rely on your fat stores.

When your diet is heavy in carbohydrates, especially the simple and refined ones like sugars and flours, your body rides that blood sugar roller coaster you learned about in the Pillar 2 chapter. If your body isn't accustomed to dipping into your fat stores between meals, you'll tend to feel sluggish. And the only way to get your energy back is to cram a bunch of sugary carbs into your mouth. It becomes a vicious cycle,

what's called a "carb adapted" system, which makes you that much more dependent on a constant flow of carbohydrates to get you through a workout, and without more carbs, you get that crash-and-burn bonk feeling.

Not good.

PreWO carbs can be helpful if you're in that mass-gain group, and a small amount—10 to 20 grams—can boost testosterone, which is necessary for muscle growth. However, unless you're a football player or a bodybuilder who's trying to get huge, preWO carbs aren't critical.

Recall that protein serves as a source of amino acids for muscle repair. Specifically, the branched-chain amino acids (BCAAs)—leucine, isoleucine, and valine—are most necessary for muscle protein synthesis. The catch is that these amino acids are essential, which means they can't be manufactured by the body and must be ingested via the food we eat. And while there is protein in plant material, the BCAAs are lacking. Therefore, if you want to repair muscle fibers, you're best off eating a protein dense in BCAAs, such as meat, poultry, seafood, or eggs.

As far as fat goes, choose one that's from healthy animal sources or plants: nuts, seeds, coconut, grass-fed butter or ghee, avocado, etc. I like coconut because it's rich in fast-burning medium-chain triglycerides (MCT), but experiment to find what works best for you.

An example of a preWO would be a hard-boiled egg (super-duper portable!) and a small handful of nuts. Or some leftover meat and a handful of olives or coconut. Or a slice of frittata. Or a protein shake with some coconut milk. Get creative.

Your Post-Workout Meal

The post-workout, or postWO, period is the thirty to sixty minutes after your exercise session ends. Recovery doesn't just come to a hard stop once an hour has passed; rather, it continues for several hours.

To get the most benefit, especially when your workout is very physically demanding and/or will happen again soon, eat as soon as you can after you finish exercising. Give yourself a chance to come back to a more parasympathetic, rest-and-digest state before trying to force food into your body, but realize that waiting a few hours isn't ideal either.

What if you're not working out hard every day? If you're including some light-to-moderate exercise in your healthy lifestyle and you're trying to improve your body composition, eating a postWO may not be necessary. You've got time between sessions to replenish your energy stores by eating your normal meals.

Pay attention to how you feel, and if you're not performing or feeling well, consider adding a postWO to the mix. On the other hand, if you're exercising several times a week or your next training session is less than twenty-four hours later, a post-workout meal matters more. It's not a substitute for a meal—you'll eat your postWO in addition to breakfast, lunch, and dinner.

Along with protein, carbohydrates are a key part of the postWO, but for a different reason than protein. Carbs help replenish the glycogen used from your muscle during your workout. If your exercise included HIIT or endurance work, you likely tapped into your glycogen stores.

Post-workout is also when you're generally more sensitive to insulin. (That's a good thing!) Eating carbohydrates causes glucose to enter the bloodstream, and then insulin is secreted from the pancreas to store the glucose away in tissues like muscle and the liver. The best type of carbohydrate for post-workout is one that's rich in glucose or starch. Add protein to your postWO, and you'll make use of increased insulin sensitivity to transport amino acids into your muscle as well.

Try to keep your postWO lower in fat. Though healthy fats are an important part of a balanced nutrition plan and they're great for helping you feel fuller longer, they slow gastric (stomach) emptying. That, in turn, slows recovery. Again, this is an important guideline to follow when your workout frequency is high because recovery speed matters more. So if you're working out hard in the evening and again in the morning, don't go crazy with fat in your post-workout meal.

If your exercise is very intense, you train back-to-back, or you've not quite recovered from your previous workout, add in a postWO and see how you do. A two-to-one ratio of carbs to protein is a good place to begin. For example, if you figure out you do best with 25 grams of protein, double that value and you'll want about 50 grams of carbohydrates. What does that look like in real food? It's roughly a chicken breast and a large white potato.

Pre- and Post-Workout Cheat Sheet

Whole sources of animal protein, carbs from starchy veggies, and healthy fats are your best options to eat before and after a workout. But when you eat matters, so use this chart to figure out the timing. Your exact needs for pre-workout will vary depending on when you ate your last meal.

	Protein	Carbs	Fats
PreWO *15 to 60 minutes before workout*	10 to 20 grams (1 to 2 ounces protein)		½ to 1 tablespoon
PostWO *Within 30 minutes after workout*	20 to 30 grams (3 to 4 ounces protein)	Double the protein grams (e.g., if 20 grams protein, then 40 grams carbs)	
EXAMPLES	Beef Eggs Fish Game Pork Poultry Protein powder Shellfish Taro Winter squash Yucca	Fruit Plantains Potato Quinoa Rice Root veggies Sweet potato Tapioca	Avocado Bacon Butter Coconut products Duck fat Grass-fed butter or ghee Olives or olive oil Nuts or nut butters Seeds Tallow

Pre-and post-workout nourishment is as much a science as it is an art. There's quite a bit of nuance to it, and rarely will one exact prescription for grams of this and grams of that work for everyone . . . or even for the same person over time.

Generally speaking, don't eat a bunch of carbs in the pre-workout period and flood your system with glucose. You should be topped up enough from the last time you trained that you don't need them. Of course, if this is a race or competition day, you want any advantage you can get, so a healthy dose of carbs before an event can help. In regular training, it's just not needed. Pre-workout, eat about two ounces protein and one tablespoon fat.

For post-workout, stick to leaner protein and starchy carbohydrates. The starchy veggies give you a lot of bang for the carb buck, but other starches like rice may work well for some people. Fruit also works, but stick to glucose-rich fruits, such as pineapple or banana, if you can. Avoid eating a lot of fat post-workout. It'll slow down digestion and therefore recovery.

Day 17 Challenge: Work Out

Note that movements from Week 2 make a dynamic warm-up. Complete all sets and reps of each movement before moving on to the next.

LEVEL 1

ALTERNATING LATERAL LUNGES—*3 sets of 6 reps with each leg*

Stand with your feet under your hips and holding a dumbbell with both hands. Step your right leg out to the side as pictured, bending your right knee and pushing your butt back. Think about sitting back into your bum by hinging at the hip instead of putting too much pressure on your knee. Your right foot should be angled slightly out, and your knee should track over your foot. Your left leg should be straight. Drive through your right foot to return to the starting position, and repeat the movement on the opposite leg.

Pro Tip

» *To make it harder,* slide the straight leg toward the bent leg to return to standing.

ALTERNATING LUNGES—*3 sets of 10 reps with each leg*

Stand with your feet under your hips, holding dumbbells in both hands. Step forward and bend your right knee to make a 90-degree angle with your right leg as you lower your left knee toward the floor. Drive through your front foot. Step forward with your left leg to bring your feet together. Repeat the movements on the opposite leg.

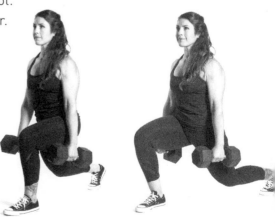

Pro Tips

» Make your step short enough that you can return to standing without swinging your torso.

» *To make it harder,* make them walking lunges, or hold the dumbbells over your head while you lunge.

ALTERNATING DUMBBELL SHOULDER PRESSES—*3 sets of 8 reps with each arm*

Stand with your feet under your hips and with dumbbells in both hands held at shoulder height, with your knuckles facing your shoulders. Engage your core, squeeze your butt, and keep your neck neutral as you actively push up through the shoulder to raise one dumbbell toward the ceiling. Keep your arm close to your head. Also, pull your ribs down instead of flaring them out. Lower the dumbbell and repeat the movements with the opposite arm.

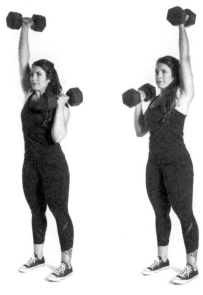

Pro Tip

» *To make it harder,* press both dumbbells up at the same time or use a barbell.

FRONT RACK CARRIES—*4 sets of 50 feet*

Stand with your feet under your hips and hold a pair of dumbbells directly in front of your chest. Engage your core and walk forward, taking normal-size steps and keeping the weights steady and close to your chest with your elbows pinned to your sides.

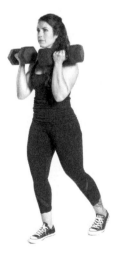

Pro Tip

» *To make it harder,* substitute a barbell for the dumbbells.

WALL SITS—*3 sets of the maximum time you can do*

Stand with your back up against a wall and your feet about a foot away from it. Slide your back down the wall until your knees are bent at 90-degree angles. Squeeze your butt, brace your abdominal muscles, and keep your neck neutral.
Hold that position as long as you can, breathing normally.

Pro Tip

» *To make it harder,* extend your arms out to your sides or overhead, or add a dumbbell to your lap.

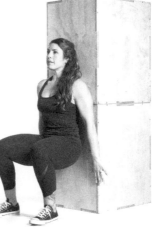

LEVEL 2

BARBELL DEADLIFTS—*1 set of 5 reps at RPE 6*

Stand with your feet under your hips with a barbell on the floor close to your shins. Hinge at the hips and grasp the barbell overhand with your hands positioned just outside your hips. Inhale, engage your core, squeeze your glutes, and push the floor away with your legs instead of lifting your back to raise the barbell.
Keep your neck neutral and the barbell close to your body as you come to a standing position, exhaling on the way up. Be sure to keep your toes from lifting off the floor throughout the movement. Hinge forward at the hips, lower the weight to the floor, and return to the starting position.

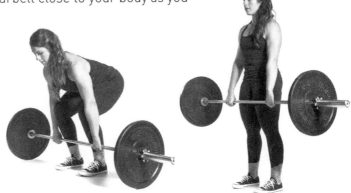

BARBELL SHOULDER PRESSES—*3 sets of 5 reps at RPE 6*

Stand with your feet under your hips and holding a barbell across the front of your shoulders with an overhand grip. Your hands should be slightly wider than shoulder width apart. Engage your core, press the barbell toward the ceiling. Maintain a neutral posture and pull your ribs down instead of flaring them out. Return to the starting position.

PULL-UPS—*4 sets of 5 reps*

Stand under a pull-up bar with your hands gripping the bar underhand or overhand (your choice) and shoulder width apart. Your thumbs should be wrapped all the way around the bar. Inhale as you engage your core and pull your body up until your chin clears the bar. Keep your neck neutral—don't crane your chin over the bar. Then lower back to the starting position with control to protect your shoulders.

Pro Tips

» *To make it easier,* secure a band around the bar and place your feet in it to reduce the amount of weight you're pulling up. Or start at the top of the pull-up position and then lower yourself down instead of doing the complete rep.

FRONT RACK CARRIES—*4 sets of 50 feet*

Stand with your feet under your hips and hold a pair of dumbbells directly in front of your chest. Engage your core and walk forward, taking normal-size steps and keeping the weights steady and close to your chest with your elbows pinned to your sides.

Pro Tip

» *To make it harder,* substitute a barbell for the dumbbells.

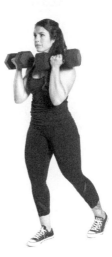

DAY 18: WHAT THE FUCK ARE YOU AFRAID OF?

Now that you know how to eat to fuel your workouts, let's explore something less concrete—and harder to get a handle on. It's fear. Merriam-Webster defines fear as "an unpleasant often strong emotion caused by anticipation or awareness of danger." And many of us walk around in fear daily.

Don't get me wrong. There are legitimate times to be afraid: when someone is threatening you with immediate harm, when you're involved in a natural disaster, when you're being chased by a wild animal. Legit fears.

Spending your time on the rocking chair of worry, though, constantly swaying back and forth in one place and never getting anywhere? Not the best use of your time or energy.

I used to worry about everything—how much fat was on my inner thighs (true story), how good (or not) of an athlete I was, what everyone was thinking about me. Sounds exhausting, right? It was. I spent so much time worrying and being afraid of "what might happen" about everything in life that I didn't have much energy left over to create and use my unique skill set to help others.

In fact, fear almost kept me from leaving a job that I was unhappy with and working on nutrition coaching full time, which, in turn, led me to develop the Core 4 program . . . and this book! I can't imagine what I'd be feeling like right now if I'd stayed in that job. But fear nearly chained me.

The thing is, when you're afraid of "what might happen" and you create fantastical scenarios in your head, you leave little space for the things you *know* you want to accomplish. That doesn't mean you need to stick your head in the sand about the realities of what life throws at you or shirk responsibility for what needs to be dealt with. You've got to step up when the time comes.

But you know what? Humans are incredibly resourceful. When the real pressure is on, when something you worried about actually happens, you'll find a way to deal with it. Really. You're resilient and intelligent.

What Do You Do When You're Scared or Worried?

Grab a piece of paper and write down the *worst* thing that could happen if this thing you're scared of occurs. Be honest. Once you acknowledge the worst case, you can stop worrying about it. You've said it. You've recognized it.

Now come up with some possible solutions. For example, "I lose my job" may be what you fear. The worst thing that could happen? "I can't pay my bills." Actions you could take: "Find a part-time job, do odd jobs, check out Craigslist, sell some things I don't need for cash, etc."

That's it. Remember, this fear you have hasn't even *happened* yet. It may never happen. But now you've acknowledged it and thought of some things you can do *if* it happens.

Okay. Now you've freed up some mental space, some time and energy that's so damn precious.

What do you do when you find yourself slipping into that worry mode? Create. Go make something. It doesn't mean you have to get out the finger paints or coloring books, but do something positive and creative with your energy. You'll be amazed by what you can come up with.

Day 18 Challenge: Complete the Face Your Fears Worksheet

Face Your Fears Worksheet

Use this worksheet to write down your three biggest fears. Then brainstorm possible solutions. Then fold up those fears and put them away.

Fear 1

How I'd Take Action

Fear 2

How I'd Take Action

Fear 3

How I'd Take Action

How did writing about your fears make you feel? When you name them and brainstorm solutions, it frees up your mind to learn, plan, ponder, and explore.

DAY 19: HOW TO CARDIO

Today's mission? To get smart about cardio.

Back in the Pillar 2 chapter I explained some of the common pitfalls of overdoing cardio. You may still be wondering why I don't provide structured cardio workouts as part of the program. Consider the common weight loss advice "Eat less and move more." It conjures up images of eating bits of lettuce on a plate coupled with long hours

of sweating it out on a treadmill. (I'm going to guess you don't get a great feeling when you visualize that.)

"Eat less and move more" can be misguided advice, because for optimal health, you need to think about the *quality* of what you eat and how you move, not just the *quantity*. Also, not everyone needs to eat less—some people already eat too little—and some people don't need to move more. Some are caught in the trap of chronic overexercising. So you see, that advice doesn't always work.

Which brings me back to cardio. Back in the 1950s, Ancel Keys's Seven Countries Study explored the connection between saturated dietary fat, cholesterol, and heart disease. His conclusions—now known to be based on misinterpreted and incomplete data—triggered a worldwide fear of fat and changes in governmental dietary policy that still echo in our society today.

Part of that fatphobia involved a shifting focus within the United States and other Western countries toward cardiovascular-type training. (Eastern countries, on the other hand, continued emphasizing strength training.)

The thing is, too much of *any* type of exercise is problematic. Too much cardio isn't health promoting. Too much strength training isn't either. But in my experience, more people are exposed to cardiovascular exercise than have experience with strength training. This is one reason why cardio isn't emphasized in this program.

If you love cardio and you do it in healthy doses—a few times a week and paired with strength training—I don't see a reason to stop. But for some people, too much cardio is stressful on the body. When mitochondria use oxygen to produce energy, free radicals—the nasties that can damage cells and DNA—are produced. Normally, the body has countermeasures—hello, antioxidants!—to neutralize these free radicals. But sometimes the system gets overwhelmed, especially when the body is under lots of stress, like exposure to environmental toxins, too much sugar, and a high level of exercise. When life stress is added, everything continues to compound.

Cardio without strength training can also present problems, especially when energy intake is too low. It results in either muscle loss or, simply, a lack of muscle gain, and metabolism takes a hit.

It's far easier to overdo long slow distance (LSD) cardio than it is to overdo strength training. If you overdo strength training, you exhaust your muscles and just can't lift anymore. But with LSD cardio, which uses different muscle fibers, you can keep going

and going and going. If you've ever had a runner's high, you're familiar with the good feelings that can accompany a long or strenuous bout of aerobic exercise. The "high" is the result of endorphins being released and binding to opioid receptors in your brain. When that happens, you feel less pain—and perhaps even euphoria. Endorphins can be released by many activities (like being in nature, eating a delicious meal, and being touched—whether sexually or platonically), but if you're starved for them, you may seek out ways to get a boost, like overexercise, drugs, or living the "wild" life. I can't determine what amount of cardio is too much for you here, but if you're pounding the pavement even when you're exhausted to get that "high," that may mean it's time to dial back or try something different, like a HIIT workout.

It's important to do what you love—because you'll keep doing it—but be smart about it at the same time.

Strength Training for Normal Humans

My husband, Z, coined the term "strength training for normal humans," and his philosophy—one that I share—is that, for optimal health, normal humans (those who don't aspire to elite levels of performance) can find a healthy way to balance exercise in their lives. The gist is simple: cardiovascular exercise is beneficial but easy to overdo. Too much can have the following effects:

Bone density may suffer, especially if the type of cardio done has little or no impact (like cycling or swimming).

Muscles that aren't used during cardio may atrophy.

Cortisol may increase.

Testosterone or estrogen may decrease.

It's harder to overdo strength training when you lift a few times a week. Strength training has the following effects:

There's a positive benefit to bone density.

Muscle volume and strength go up.

Testosterone and estrogen normalize.

Cortisol rises temporarily, but not to an unhealthy level given adequate recovery.

A few strength-training sessions per week is enough to give you all those benefits. Yet I truly believe you should never do something you hate, even if it's "healthy." In fact, research shows that you're more likely to stick to healthy eating or exercise when you choose foods and activities you enjoy.

If, at the end of the program, you really don't think strength training has a place in your life, at least you gave it a fair shake. But I hope that if you do return to high-volume cardio, you'll blend strength training into your routine once or twice a week in order to enjoy some of its benefits.

Day 19 Challenge: Work Out

Note that movements from Week 2 make a great dynamic warm-up. Complete all sets and reps of each movement before moving on to the next.

LEVEL 1

GOBLET SQUATS—*4 sets of 10 reps*

Stand with your feet slightly wider than hip width and hold a dumbbell or kettlebell in front of your chest. Inhale and engage your core as you hinge from your hips and bend your knees to lower your bottom toward the floor, keeping your feet in a comfortable squat stance with your thighs a little lower than parallel. Exhale as you return to the starting position.

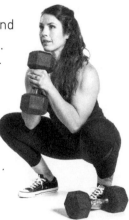

SUITCASE DEADLIFTS—*4 sets of 10 reps*

Position your feet hip width apart and hold dumbbells or kettlebells next to your feet. Engage your core, squeeze your glutes, and come to a standing position by trying to push the floor away with your legs instead of lifting with your back. Keep your neck neutral throughout the movement, and keep the weights close to your body. Then hinge forward at the hip and return to the starting position. Be sure to keep your toes from lifting off the floor throughout the movement.

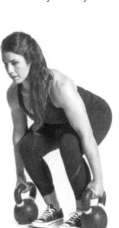

Pro Tip

» *To make it harder,* use a barbell.

RENEGADE ROWS—*3 sets of 10 reps*

Lie facedown on the floor with dumbbells on either side of your body at about chest level. While grasping the dumbbells, push your body up into a plank position. Shift your weight onto your right arm and bend your left arm to row that dumbbell up to the left side of your rib cage. Actively pull with the upper back into each row, keeping the arm close to your body. Lower the dumbbell to the floor and repeat the movements with the other arm.

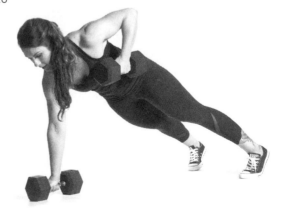

PULL-UPS—*4 sets of 6 reps*

Stand under a pull-up bar with your hands gripping the bar underhand or overhand (your choice) and shoulder width apart. Your thumbs should be wrapped all the way around the bar. Inhale as you engage your core and pull your body up until your chin clears the bar. Keep your neck neutral—don't crane your chin over the bar. Then lower back to the starting position with control to protect your shoulders.

Pro Tips

» *To make it easier,* secure a band around the bar and place your feet in it to reduce the amount of weight you're pulling up. Or start at the top of the pull-up position and then lower yourself down instead of doing the complete rep.

L SITS—*3 sets*

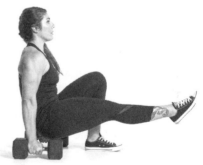

Sit on the floor with your legs extended in front of you and your hands gripping dumbbells on the floor next to your hips. Inhale and engage your core as you lift your butt off the floor, supporting your bodyweight on your hands. Hold for 15 to 30 seconds, then lower to the floor.

Pro Tip

» *To make it easier,* lift one leg off the floor—it can be either bent or straight.

LEVEL 2

BARBELL BACK SQUATS—*5 sets of 3 reps at RPE 6*

Stand with a barbell resting across the meaty back of your shoulders, called the trapezius muscles, and held in an overhand grip. Don't let the barbell rest on your neck bones. Inhale, engage your core, squeeze your glutes, and hinge at the hip before bending your knees to lower your butt toward the floor until your thighs are parallel to the floor or slightly lower. Keep your neck neutral and your chest high, then return to the starting position, exhaling on the way up.

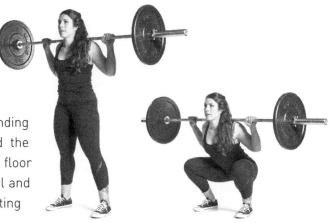

BARBELL POWER CLEANS—*3 sets of 2 reps at RPE 7*

Stand with your feet slightly wider than hip width apart and with a barbell on the floor in front of your feet. Hinge at the hips and grab the barbell overhand with your hands positioned just outside your hips. Lift it to your thighs, then push with your legs and jump as you bend your elbows to flip the bar up and shrug it to your shoulders. The power comes from your legs driving the bar up rather than pulling it with your arms. Stand in a partial squat with your knees slightly bent. Pause briefly, then return the bar to the floor.

Pro Tip

» *To make it harder,* use an unbalanced object like a sandbag, or receive the weight in a full squat clean.

L SITS—*3 sets*

Sit on the floor with your legs extended in front of you and your hands gripping dumbbells on the floor next to your hips. Inhale and engage your core as you lift your butt off the floor, supporting your bodyweight on your hands. Hold for 15 to 30 seconds, then lower to the floor.

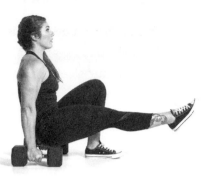

Pro Tip

» *To make it easier,* lift one leg off the floor—it can be either bent or straight.

PUSH-UPS—*4 sets of 5 reps*

Lie facedown on the floor and place your hands on the floor next to your body at about chest level, with your elbows close to your sides. Your body should look like an arrow if you could view it from above, not the letter T. Push your body up so that you're on your hands and toes, keeping your body in a straight line. Don't stick your butt up into the air or drop your butt too low. Bend your elbows to lower your chest toward the floor, and then push back up. As you push up, take a breath and keep your butt and core tight.

Pro Tip

» *To make it harder,* add weight on your back, or try clapping push-ups.

DAY 20: SLEEP, PART 2

Today's challenge may surprise you, and you aren't experiencing déjà vu. We're gonna talk about sleep . . . again. Earlier in the program, you saw why sleep is totes important. You tracked your sleep for a week to get insight and perhaps find patterns. Today, let's consider how you can fall asleep faster and look at some other practical tips for sleeping better.

Five Ways to Fall Asleep Faster

1. MAKE A BEDTIME ROUTINE.

We create bedtime routines for children, but we tend to shun them as adults. By following the same routines around bedtime, you're training yourself that it's time to wind down and sleep.

What does this look like? It's totally up to you, but make it low-stress and relaxing. Maybe you read for a while, then set out your work clothes for the next day, take a shower, and brush your teeth. Build repetition so you know that at the end of the routine, it's time to sleep.

Even more important than that is going to sleep and waking at roughly the same time. Erratic bedtimes make it hard to train your body and brain to prepare for sleep.

2. TAKE MAGNESIUM BEFORE BED.

Magnesium is a vital mineral for hundreds of biochemical reactions in the body, including muscle function, electrolyte balance, cellular energy production, and more. Also, it helps with a feeling of relaxation, so it's great to take before bedtime.

Good dietary sources include dark leafy greens, sea vegetables, and nuts. Interestingly, some minerals, such as calcium, may compete with magnesium for absorption, so avoid having large amounts of calcium-rich foods at the same time.

You might also try a relaxing Epsom salt bath or using magnesium oil on your skin.

Aim to take your magnesium about thirty minutes before bedtime.

3. USE LAVENDER OIL.

Lavender is renowned for its ability to calm and relax the body, and it makes a great addition to your bedtime routine. Here are some ways to use lavender oil for better sleep:

> Add lavender oil to your Epsom salt bath (be careful because it can make the bathtub slippery).
>
> Mix a few drops in a spray bottle with water and mist your sheets and bedding.
>
> Put a drop or two on your temples or on the bottoms of your feet.
>
> Diffuse lavender oil while you sleep.

Lavender essential oil is generally safe to apply undiluted, but check for skin sensitivities before using it, especially on large areas of skin. Or dilute it in a carrier oil, such as coconut oil.

4. AVOID NIGHTTIME BLUE LIGHT.

This. Is. Huge.

As you learned in the Pillar 3 chapter, nighttime exposure to light, particularly the blue wavelengths that mimic sunlight, is incredibly disruptive to melatonin, the hormone that helps put you to sleep. Unfortunately, the backlit electronic devices that are so prevalent in our modern world are oozing with blue light.

Daytime exposure to blue wavelengths is important because it helps maintain the "awake" part of your circadian rhythm. However, reducing or avoiding blue light once the sun goes down is key to falling asleep faster.

To cut down on nighttime blue light:

> Use screen dimmers such as Night Shift or f.lux on your electronic devices. These programs turn your screens to a yellow-orange hue, mimicking sunset and candlelight. Better yet, avoid screens for an hour or two before bed.
>
> Wear amber glasses, also known as "blue blockers." They may look nerdy, but these orange-lens glasses filter some of the blue light coming from your

screens. At ten dollars a pair for the generic kind, that's a pretty inexpensive solution to help you feel less stimulated at night. You can get fancy ones for a little more money.

Eliminate light sources in your bedroom, such as digital alarm clocks, electronic devices with glowing power lights, and ambient light coming through your windows. Blackout curtains are a must.

Use salt lamps or incandescent bulbs on a dimmer for soft light sources that don't throw blue light and aren't as dangerous as candles.

5. REDUCE STRESS, ESPECIALLY IN THE EVENING.

Okay, it's hard to eliminate 100 percent of stress from your life. I get that. But night-time stress can make it particularly hard to fall asleep.

The hormone cortisol is associated with a healthy circadian rhythm; it ramps up as morning approaches and peaks by midmorning, helping you wake up and stay alert. When cortisol rises at night, though, it can make you feel too keyed up to wind down.

Psychological stress is the type we often think of, but physical stress—especially from evening workout sessions—can also make it difficult to fall asleep. If you train in the evening and are having trouble sleeping, you may want to switch your exercise schedule.

To reduce evening stress, also try to

do some light stretching or yoga;

practice deep breathing or meditation;

avoid suspenseful or physiologically thrilling books and TV programs in the evening;

stay off work email and social media so you don't get stressed out; and/or

read a book or take a warm bath or shower.

In addition to these five strategies, a healthy diet rich in nutrient-dense foods (what you're eating this month) is the best foundation for balancing the hormones responsible for your circadian rhythm and sleep. Try to implement these suggestions before

turning to pharmaceutical intervention. If you continue to suffer from sleep issues, seek the help of a health professional.

Day 20 Challenge: Include Sleep Strategies

Pick one or two of the sleep strategies just mentioned and start doing them tonight.

OPTIONAL WEEKEND WORKOUT. Do some interval training, resting 90 seconds between each interval. You might try one of these:

> Run—100 meters, 5 to 7 sets
>
> Row—250 meters, 5 to 7 sets
>
> Stationary bike—30 seconds, 5 to 7 sets
>
> Swim—25 meters, 5 to 7 sets

DAY 21: EATING OUT WITHOUT "CHEATING"

I hope you slept like a proverbial baby last night—a baby who wakes up rested and refreshed and ready to kick ass and take names. Today's challenge is easy peasy, so get ready: prep your meals for the week ahead. By now it should be getting easier for sure, and you may be ready to make some tweaks. Remember, it's all about developing habits that will set you up for success each week.

You've got this! Go prep your little heart out! And while we're on the subject of food, let's talk about dining out.

How to Eat Out—Without Going Crazy

Staying at home for the rest of your life because you're unsure about how to navigate a restaurant menu is no fun. You're cultivating better choices for the long term, so after this program, it will be up to you to take the wheel.

One of the areas where you may struggle is how to go out to eat without ordering (and eating) allthefoodsanddrinks. But it's inevitable that you'll eat out from time to time. When it becomes a daily thing because "I didn't meal prep and my fridge is bare

and, oh look, how did that giant plate of greasy food end up in front of me *again* . . . ?!" that's when there could be a problem.

However, many restaurants are becoming more accommodating. A lot of them have healthier options or are willing to make substitutions to dishes if you ask. Every once in a while I run across a place unable to meet my request, but I find it's rare, as long as it's a reasonable ask.

I try not to sweat stuff like what kind of oil they used to sauté my veggies in. If you start analyzing everything to that degree, you're missing out on the joy of having someone else cook your food (and do the damn dishes). Don't end up with analysis paralysis.

Tips for Eating Out

Here are some tips to help you make healthier choices when eating out:

Ask about a gluten-free menu or items if you're gluten sensitive.

Skip deep-fried foods.

Tell the waitperson to hold the breadbasket.

Omit the bun or bread from a burger and ask for a lettuce wrap or a side salad instead.

Request to substitute extra veggies or a potato for fries.

Ask for dressing or sauce on the side.

Look for simple dishes, like a meat entrée with veggies on the side, instead of casseroles or fried items that tend to be higher in calories.

Skip the dessert menu. (Some restaurants are so special that it may be worth having dessert, but at a chain restaurant, that's probably not the case.)

Pass up alcohol. Sparkling water with lemon is a nice fizzy drink instead of booze.

Day 21 Challenge: Prep Meals for Next Week

See the beginning of the next chapter for the upcoming week's shopping list and what to prep.

Finish Strong

Oh heck yes, you have arrived at Week 4! If you don't often stop to take stock of what you've accomplished, now is the time to give yourself a pat on the back for staying committed and continuing to show up and take action. You've achieved more than a lot of people ever will, because it's one thing to wish for change and quite another thing to make it happen. I know the big sexy payoff moments are exciting, but if you can recognize the subtle—but powerful—shifts you're making, that's huge, too.

You have so many new tools and experiences in your toolbox going into this last week of the Core 4 program. Remember to dip into the resources to keep shaping your nourishing food plan, workouts, restful moments, and mindset. Finish out this month strong!

Week 4 Shopping List

Bacon (8 ounces
   plus 4 slices)
Cheddar cheese, shredded
   full-fat (10 ounces),
   optional

Chicken breast
   (1 pound)
Chicken sausage, any flavor
   (1 pound)
Eggs (19)

Ground beef (3½ pounds)
Pork breakfast sausage
   (12 ounces)
Salmon (1½ pounds)
Sirloin steak (1 pound)

Avocados (4)

Bananas (3)

Basil leaves, fresh (3 cups)

Blueberries (1 pint)

Broccoli (1 pound)

Carrot (1)

Cauliflower (4 pounds)

Cherry tomatoes (1 pint)

Cilantro, fresh (1 bunch)
    + Cilantro, fresh
    (1 bunch), optional

Cucumber (1)

Fingerling potatoes
    (12 ounces)

Garlic (8 cloves)

Ginger, fresh (1 inch)

Green beans (8 ounces)

Green leaf lettuce (1 head)

Green onions (3)

Jicama (1)

Kale (4 bunches)

Lemons (2)

Limes (8 to 9)

Mint, fresh (1 bunch)

Napa cabbage (1)

Parsley, fresh (1 bunch)

Poblano pepper (1)

Red bell pepper (1)

Red cabbage (1)

Roma tomatoes (3 plus
    2 pounds)

Shallot (1)

Spinach (1 8-ounce bag)

Sweet onion (1)

Sweet potatoes (3 plus
    2 pounds)

Swiss chard (1 bunch)

Thyme, fresh (4 to 6 sprigs)

Yukon gold potatoes
    (1 pound)

Almond milk (1¼ cup plus
    1 tablespoon)

Almonds, chopped (¼ cup)

Ancho chili powder
    (3 teaspoons)

Avocado oil mayonnaise
    (¼ cup)

Balsamic vinegar (⅓ cup)

Black olives, sliced (¼ cup)

Chia seeds (2 tablespoons)

Chicken broth, low-sodium
    (1 cup)

Chipotle pepper, ground
    (¼ teaspoon)

Cinnamon, ground
    (2 teaspoons)

Coconut aminos
    (4 teaspoons)

Coconut milk (16 ounces)

Coconut, shredded and
    unsweetened (1 cup)

Collagen powder
    (2 tablespoons), optional

Cumin, ground (½ teaspoon)

Currants, dried, or raisins
    (2 tablespoons)

Dark sesame oil (1 teaspoon)

Extra-virgin olive oil or ghee

Fish sauce (¾ teaspoon)

Flaxseed, ground (½ cup)

Garlic powder
    (¾ teaspoons)

Harissa sauce, mild
    (2 tablespoons)

Hemp hearts
    (2 tablespoons)

Medjool dates (2)

Onion powder (½ teaspoon)

Oregano, dried (¼ teaspoon)

Parsley, dried (½ teaspoon)

Pickled jalapeño rings
    (1 tablespoon), optional

Pine nuts (¼ cup)

Pistachios, shelled (½ cup)

Rice noodles
    (1 8-ounce package)

Rice wine vinegar
    (2 teaspoons)

Salt and pepper

Smoked paprika
    (½ teaspoon)

Taco seasoning
    (2 tablespoons)

Tahini (1 tablespoon)

Tart cherries, dried (½ cup)

Thyme, dried (¼ teaspoon)

Tortilla chips, grain-free
    (6 ounces)

Vanilla extract (3 teaspoons)

DAY 21

For this day's breakfast, lunch, and dinner eat leftovers from the previous week.

Meals to prep:

- » Sweet Potato Breakfast Bowls (page 262)
- » Roasted Tomato and Garlic Soup (page 263)
- » Fresh Spring Roll Salad with Ginger-Lime Dressing (page 266), dressing stored on the side
- » Pesto Salmon Sheet Tray Bake (page 284)

Other prep:

- » 1 bunch swiss chard, steam
- » 2 pounds cauliflower, roast

DAY 22

BREAKFAST: Sweet Potato Breakfast Bowls + steamed swiss chard

LUNCH: Fresh Spring Roll Salad with Ginger-Lime Dressing

DINNER: Pesto Salmon Sheet Tray Bake + Roasted Tomato and Garlic Soup

DAY 23

BREAKFAST: Sweet Potato Breakfast Bowls + roasted cauliflower

LUNCH: Pesto Salmon Sheet Tray Bake + Roasted Tomato and Garlic Soup

DINNER: Fresh Spring Roll Salad with Ginger-Lime Dressing

DAY 24

BREAKFAST: Sweet Potato Breakfast Bowls + steamed swiss chard

LUNCH: Fresh Spring Roll Salad with Ginger-Lime Dressing

DINNER: Pesto Salmon Sheet Tray Bake + roasted cauliflower

DAY 25

BREAKFAST: Savory Ham and Egg Cups + steamed swiss chard

LUNCH: Roasted Tomato and Garlic Soup + roasted cauliflower

DINNER: Loaded Taco Beef Nachos with Avocado Crema (prepare today)

Meals to prep:

» Breakfast Sausage Casserole (page 257)

» Sautéed Kale with Balsamic Cherries (page 272)

» Loaded Taco Beef Nachos with Avocado Crema (page 276)

Other prep:

» 1 8-ounce bag fresh spinach, steam

» 1 pound chicken sausage, cook

DAY 26

BREAKFAST: Breakfast Sausage Casserole + steamed spinach

LUNCH: Chicken sausage + Sautéed Kale with Balsamic Cherries

DINNER: Loaded Taco Beef Nachos with Avocado Crema

DAY 27

BREAKFAST: Breakfast Sausage Casserole + steamed spinach

LUNCH: Loaded Taco Beef Nachos with Avocado Crema

DINNER: Chicken sausage + Sautéed Kale with Balsamic Cherries

DAY 28

For this day's breakfast, lunch, and dinner, eat leftovers from the previous week.

Meals to prep:

» Mini Meatloaf Sheet Tray Bake (page 277)

» Steak Cobb Salad with Southwestern Ranch Dressing (page 267), dressing stored on the side

» Banana Cinnamon No-Oatmeal (page 260)

» The Best Cauliflower Ever (page 273)

Other prep:

» 2 bunches kale, steam

DAY 29

BREAKFAST: Banana Cinnamon No-Oatmeal + steamed kale

LUNCH: Steak Cobb Salad with Southwestern Ranch Dressing

DINNER: Mini Meatloaf Sheet Tray Bake + The Best Cauliflower Ever

DAY 30

BREAKFAST: Banana Cinnamon No-Oatmeal + steamed kale

LUNCH: Steak Cobb Salad with Southwestern Ranch Dressing

DINNER: Mini Meatloaf Sheet Tray Bake + The Best Cauliflower Ever

DAY 22: THE 90-30 WORKFLOW

Earlier in the program, on Day 14, you learned about how humans aren't machines: our energy needs replenishing throughout the day. Inside your daily circadian rhythm, you have the shorter ultradian rhythm. If you've ever struggled to push through a long

workday and stay highly motivated, focused, and attentive all the way through, you're not alone. And if you multitask all day only to wind up feeling like you're exhausted but like you accomplished nothing, you're not alone either.

These two methods of working aren't just common—they're often baked right into workplace culture. A friend of mine started a job at a biotech company and was dismayed that though the workday ended at 5:00 p.m., his coworkers were all anxious to take advantage of overtime hours. It was an unwritten expectation that, as a team player, he stay longer. (And longer. And longer.)

Even if you work from home or have more flexibility in your schedule, how often do you take breaks? During your breaks, do you engage in activities that leave you recharged? And if your workplace culture or the shifts you work don't allow for frequent breaks, do you make the most out of the time you *do* get?

Contrary to popular belief, pushing through very long blocks of work time doesn't result in higher productivity. The opposite is true. And more surprising, even very short—but meaningful—breaks can leave you feeling refreshed, energized, and ready to focus again.

Implementing the 90-30 Workflow

In order to get more frequent, renewing breaks in my day, I adopted the 90-30 workflow, which I detailed in the Pillar 3 chapter (page 67). If you'll recall, the idea is that for every 90 minutes of focused work time, you take a 30-minute renewal break.

The 30-minute break can be something active or passive, such as eating a meal, walking, reading a book, exercising, or meditating. The key is to avoid habits that further drain your energy.

What each person finds revitalizing will vary. But be honest: checking your email or social media on your break isn't necessarily recharging. And if you can't break every 90 minutes because of your schedule, just focus on working in the time chunks you can, then doing something renewing on your break. I sometimes take a pause every half hour to stretch my legs or give my eyes a screen break.

Then I repeat the 90-minute block. When I get back into my block, I use a couple of things to help get into work mode: I sign out of social media, put on noise-canceling headphones, and set a timer on my phone or computer. These little rituals signify that

it's time to focus and get down to business. It's *amazing* how much more work I get done in a shorter period of time.

As I also mentioned earlier, I recommend doing about four of these cycles in one workday if you can, though I know that's not always possible for everyone. When you build more downtime into your day, you'll not only get more done but feel better at the end of the day too. How's that for rad?!

Day 22 Challenge: Practice at Least One 90-30 Cycle, plus Work Out

Exercises from Week 3 make great warm-up moves. Complete all sets and reps of each movement before moving on to the next.

LEVEL 1

STEP-UPS—*4 sets of 8 reps with each leg*

Stand next to a sturdy box or weight bench. Step your left foot onto the box or bench, and drive through your forward foot as you lift your right foot up to meet your left. Step down carefully with your left foot first—don't jump down—and do all reps with your left foot first before repeating the movements with the other foot.

Pro Tip

» *To make it harder,* hold dumbbells in your hands, or substitute box jumps—step down carefully!

SINGLE-LEG DEADLIFTS—*3 sets of 8 reps with each leg*

Stand with your feet hip width apart and with dumbbells in both hands. Engage your core and keep your spine aligned as you shift your weight onto your left foot. Hinge forward at the hip to lower the weights until they reach the middle of your left shin as you extend your right leg behind you, balancing on your left. Feel your glute and hamstring on the standing leg activate, and soften the standing knee—don't lock it. Keep your hips square. Rise back to the standing position and do all the reps before switching legs and repeating the movements.

Pro Tip

» *To make it easier,* do this move without dumbbells and put one hand on a wall to keep your balance.

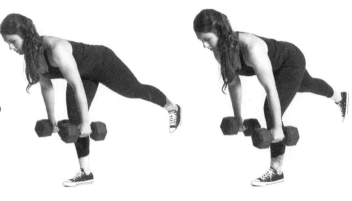

ALTERNATING BICEPS CURLS—*4 sets of 10 reps with each arm*

Stand with your feet under your hips and hold dumbbells in your hands (as pictured). Engage your core and keep your spine aligned as you bend your right arm to bring the dumbbell up to your shoulder. Keep your elbow close to your side. Then lower your right arm. Repeat the movement with the left arm.

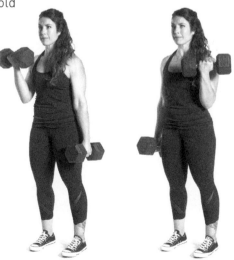

Pro Tip

» *To make it harder,* curl both dumbbells up at the same time instead of alternating.

SEATED SIDE TWISTS—*3 sets of 10 reps on each side*

Sit on the floor with your knees bent, your feet flat on the floor, and a dumbbell held in both hands at chest height. Lean back, bringing your feet off the floor, and slowly twist your body to the right as you move the dumbbell toward your right hip. Keep your sit bones on the floor. Then rotate your body slowly to the left, moving the dumbbell toward your left hip. Keep the weight close to your body as you rotate from side to side.

SUPER(WO)MANS OR BIRD DOGS—*4 sets of 10 reps*

Lie facedown on the floor and extend your arms out in front of you. Engage your core and lift your arms and legs a few inches off the floor. Activate your back and butt muscles, moving slowly until you reach a comfortable maximum height. Hold for 1 to 3 seconds, then return to the starting position.

Pro Tips

» *To make it harder,* increase the reps.

» *To make it easier,* decrease the reps, or don't lift as far off the floor. You can also substitute with bird dogs: position yourself on all fours on the floor and extend one arm out in front of you while also extending the opposite leg out behind you, keeping your weight centered; then switch the arm and leg.

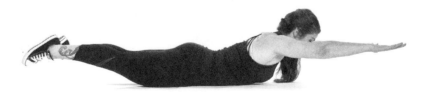

LEVEL 2

BARBELL BACK SQUATS—*5 sets of 5 reps at RPE 7*

Stand with a barbell resting across the meaty back of your shoulders, called the trapezius muscles, and held in an overhand grip. Don't let the barbell rest on your neck bones. Inhale, engage your core, squeeze your glutes, and hinge at the hip before bending your knees to lower your butt toward the floor until your thighs are parallel to the floor or slightly lower. Keep your neck neutral and your chest high, then return to the starting position, exhaling on the way up.

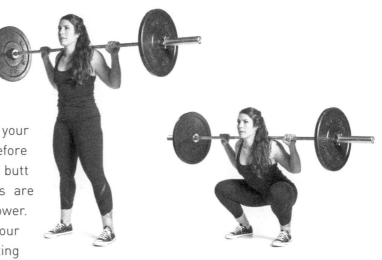

BARBELL SHOULDER PRESSES—*3 sets of 5 reps at RPE 6*

Stand with your feet under your hips and holding a barbell across the front of your shoulders with an overhand grip. Your hands should be slightly wider than shoulder width apart. Engage your core and press the barbell toward the ceiling. Maintain a neutral posture and pull your ribs down instead of flaring them out. Return to the starting position.

PULL-UPS —*4 sets of 5 or more reps*

Stand under a pull-up bar with your hands gripping the bar underhand or overhand (your choice) and shoulder width apart. Your thumbs should be wrapped all the way around the bar. Inhale as you engage your core and pull your body up until your chin clears the bar. Keep your neck neutral—don't crane your chin over the bar. Then lower back to the starting position with control to protect your shoulders.

Pro Tips

» *To make it easier,* secure a band around the bar and place your feet in it to reduce the amount of weight you're pulling up. Or start at the top of the pull-up position and then lower yourself down instead of doing the complete rep.

WINDMILLS —*3 sets of 10 reps on each side*

Stand with your feet slightly wider than hip width apart and with your arms extended out to your sides at shoulder height. Engage your core and twist your body to bring your right hand toward your left foot. Return to the starting position, upright, and then twist your body to the left, bringing your left hand toward your right foot. Return again to the starting position and repeat.

Pro Tip

» *To make this harder,* hold a light dumbbell in the hand that's overhead. Do all the reps on one side before switching the dumbbell to the other hand and doing the reps on the other side.

DAY 23: MODERATION

There's a famous saying: "Everything in moderation."

This phrase is tricky for a few reasons, the most important of which is that some things, in moderation, are super unhealthy or can cause disease, allergic reaction, or even death. I know it's an attempt to sum up a philosophy on life, but it really comes down to you. Is [insert anything] in moderation a good idea *for you*? For example, what if you have celiac disease? Any amount of gluten in your diet will seriously impact your health.

Always consider *your* goals, needs, and context when playing with the idea of moderation.

Some of my clients identify themselves as moderators, those who live by the "Everything in moderation" philosophy, while others avoid certain foods, drinks, habits, or behaviors 100 percent of the time. For example, I abstain from alcohol, but I'm a moderator when it comes to chocolate. (A square or two of dark chocolate is usually all I need to feel satisfied.) You might have the opposite consumption habit and be a moderator when it comes to alcohol but abstain from chocolate. Or maybe you moderate both . . . or abstain from both.

This is where things get tricky.

Willpower Versus Inner Power

There's a difference, energetically, between avoiding something because it's the only way to control yourself and *choosing* to avoid it because it makes you feel less good. I know it's technically the same thing at the end of the day—you just don't eat or drink or do that thing—but the effect it has on your willpower and energy is undeniable. The former is more draining and disempowering. The latter is owning your choices, and that's inner power.

If you avoid certain foods not because they make you sick or make you feel less than good, be very clear about why. Here's an example: one of my clients did everything in her power to never eat french fries. She believed they were bad for her—an off-limits food—because she felt she couldn't control herself. She decided that if she couldn't eat a whole order of fries, then it was better to never eat a single one.

Every time she went out to eat with friends and saw them order french fries, a back-and-forth dialogue went through her mind. She'd spend the whole meal thinking about fries.

When she got home—particularly if her day had been stressful—she'd order take-out and almost always follow it up with overdoing it on something sugary before bed. I finally asked her, "What would happen if you let yourself get french fries? Could you eat a few and be satisfied?"

"Yes," she admitted, "but I'd be afraid I'd eat all of them." From there I asked her to get clear about her fear. It all pointed back to her not trusting herself to stop. She ended up in a mental tug of war, which then used up her willpower and left her feeling more stressed. In this state of mind, she almost invariably overdid it with other "bad" food.

And if she ate them all, we reframed it: She didn't go out to eat every day and order french fries at every meal. She could own her choice and move on.

She ultimately ordered the fries, ate about half, and stopped eating. Plus, she didn't go home and overdo it that night. The wonderful part was that she lost the mental anguish and shameful self-talk, and she mindfully made the best choice for her in that moment. She finally felt empowered to make decisions about food for herself.

I'm not saying that you need to flip-flop on everything you've ever done. My hope is that you'll take a look with more awareness of what's driving your decisions. Are you coming from a place of love and compassion for yourself? Or is your reaction motivated by fear?

Food for thought.

Day 23 Challenge: Journal Your Answers to These Questions

What foods do you moderate?

What foods do you avoid?

What role, if any, does fear play in the things you avoid eating?

DAY 24: PERFECTLY IMPERFECT

I want to mention a hot topic in the fitness world: body perfection.

My weight has fluctuated quite a bit in my adult life. I was at my lowest weight when I was an Xterra athlete, doing a ton of endurance mountain biking and not eating enough, but I still wasn't happy with my body because I wasn't "thin enough" in my own eyes. The point is, as you can imagine, my happiness was not actually tied to my bodyweight because I could not be satisfied no matter how small I got.

When I found weight training through CrossFit in 2010, things significantly changed for me. I put on muscle mass and got a whole helluva lot stronger. I'd already been eating better for six months, and my health was improving. And even though I was "bigger," I didn't hate my body anymore. Why? I shifted my focus to health and the amazing things my body could do instead of reaching an exact scale weight.

I've come to appreciate my capable body, and it's my hope that the same will happen for you. You don't have to have a six-pack or be 10 percent body fat to have worth as a person.

In other words: *Your worth is not found in your physical body, despite what society says.*

So, yes, I love my thick thighs . . . even if they make finding pants a challenging task sometimes.

Please take some time to think about whether your aspirations for your physical body are realistic, safe, healthy, and/or worth the time and sacrifice they'll take to achieve. If, for example, you're pouring a huge amount of time, energy, and self-deprivation into seeing your abs, honestly evaluate the trade-off. Is the cost worth the benefit? Is it giving you more than it's taking from you? Both important questions.

Day 24 Challenge: Work Out

Movements from last week make a great dynamic warm-up. Complete all sets and reps of each movement before moving on to the next.

Squat Mobilization

Hopefully you've been finding some new favorite mobility drills to target stiff areas of your body before you work out.

Let's talk about my favorite squat mobility drill: hip openers. Yes, squats demand mobility in several areas of your body, from your ankles up to your thoracic spine. But perhaps the area that takes the most heat from regular squatting (and sitting) is the hip area. The glutes, hip flexors, and hamstrings can end up tight, overused, or imbalanced.

If you haven't tried these two yet, incorporate them before your workout today:

GLUTE MASSAGE: Take a lacrosse ball or softball and position it under one of your glutes, right in the meaty butt cheek. Search for a tight spot. Then lean a bent knee over outside the hips to the left or right. Do this several times. You can even move the lacrosse ball toward the outer part of the hip. Your butt cheek will feel softer instead of tense and knotted.

SITTING HIP MOBILIZATION (GREAT TO DO AT YOUR DESK DURING THE DAY!): Sit in a chair and cross your left foot over your right knee so your shin is parallel with the floor. Fold slightly forward. You can keep the left foot from sliding off your knee by holding it down with your hand. Gently push your left knee down.

GLUTE BRIDGES—*4 sets of 10 reps*

Lie on your back with your knees bent, your feet flat on the floor and close to your hips, and your arms at your sides on the floor. Engage your core and squeeze your butt as you slowly drive your hips up toward the ceiling so that your body is in a straight line from head to knees. Keep your knees parallel to each other; don't let them collapse in or out. Slowly lower your hips back to the starting position.

Pro Tip

» *To make it harder*, lift up one leg at a time from the bridge position.

SPLIT SQUATS—*4 sets of 10 reps with each leg*

Stand with your feet under your hips and with dumbbells held at shoulder height. Step forward with your left leg into a lunge stance. Engage your core and gently lower your right knee toward the floor until both legs form 90-degree angles. Return to a standing position, then lower your right knee again. Do all reps on this leg before driving through your front foot, engaging your glutes, and returning to the starting position. Repeat with opposite leg positions.

Pro Tip

» *To make it harder*, place your back foot up on a bench (to do a Bulgarian split squat).

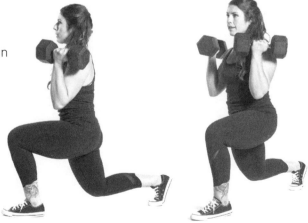

ALTERNATING DUMBBELL ROWS—*4 sets of 8 reps with each arm*

Holding a dumbbell in your left hand, to begin with, stand with your right foot forward in a partial lunge and your body from your left heel to the top of your head forming almost a straight line. Keep your abs engaged, your spine aligned, and your elbow close to your body as you pull the dumbbell up to your ribs, then lower it. You can rest your other hand on your knee or your leg for support. Repeat the movements on the opposite side.

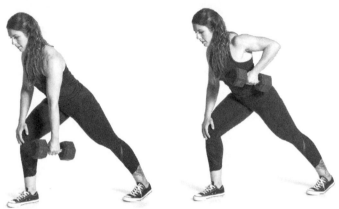

DIPS—*3 sets of 6 to 8 reps*

Sit on a sturdy bench or box with your hands next to you and your feet about twelve inches in front of your hips. Slide your bum off the bench, and keeping your body close to the bench, bend your arms to slowly lower your body a few inches below the bench, then drive back up, using your triceps, to the starting position.

Pro Tips

» *To make it easier,* set your feet closer to your body.

» *To make it harder,* set your feet farther from your body.

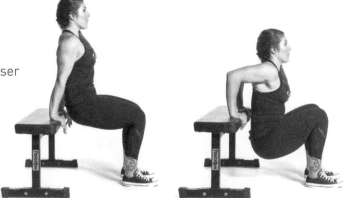

WAITER WALKS—*4 sets of 50 feet with each arm*

Stand with your feet under your hips and hold light- to moderate-weight dumbbells in each hand. Press your right dumbbell up toward the ceiling, actively pushing through your shoulder and keeping your right arm close to your head. Then walk with the dumbbell overhead. Pull your ribs down instead of flaring them out. Repeat the movements with your left arm.

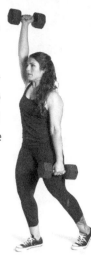

LEVEL 2

BARBELL DEADLIFTS—*1 set of 5 reps at RPE 7*

Stand with your feet under your hips with a barbell on the floor close to your shins. Hinge at the hips and grasp the barbell overhand with your hands positioned just outside your hips. Inhale, engage your core, squeeze your glutes, and push the floor away with your legs instead of lifting your back to raise the barbell. Keep your neck neutral and the barbell close to your body as you come to a standing position, exhaling on the way up. Be sure to keep your toes from lifting off the floor throughout the movement. Hinge forward at the hips, lower the weight to the floor, and return to the starting position.

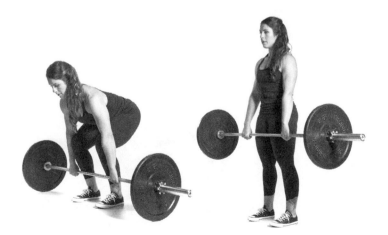

BARBELL POWER CLEANS—*3 sets of 2 reps at RPE 7*

Stand with your feet slightly wider than hip width apart and with a barbell on the floor in front of your feet. Hinge at the hips and grab the barbell overhand with your hands positioned just outside your hips. Lift it to your thighs, then push with your legs and jump as you bend your elbows to flip the bar up and shrug it to your shoulders. The power comes from your legs driving the bar up rather than pulling it with your arms. Stand in a partial squat with your knees slightly bent. Pause briefly, then return the bar to the floor.

Pro Tip

» *To make it harder,* use an unbalanced object like a sandbag, or receive the weight in a full squat clean.

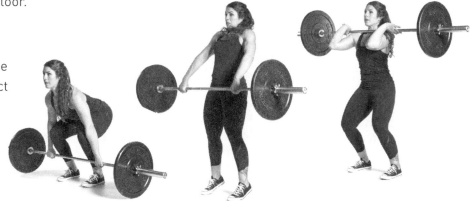

PUSH-UPS—*4 sets of 5 or more reps*

Lie facedown on the floor and place your hands on the floor next to your body at about chest level, with your elbows close to your sides. Your body should look like an arrow if you could view it from above, not the letter T. Push your body up so that you're on your hands and toes, keeping your body in a straight line. Don't stick your butt up into the air or drop your butt too low. Bend your elbows to lower your chest toward the floor, and then push back up. As you push up, take a breath and keep your butt and core tight.

Pro Tip

» *To make it harder,* add weight on your back, or try clapping push-ups.

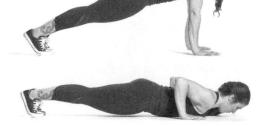

SUPER(WO)MANS OR BIRD DOGS—*4 sets of 10 reps*

Lie facedown on the floor and extend your arms out in front of you. Engage your core and lift your arms and legs a few inches off the floor. Activate your back and butt muscles, moving slowly until you reach a comfortable maximum height. Hold for 1 to 3 seconds, then return to the starting position.

Pro Tips

» *To make it harder,* increase the reps.

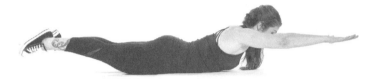

» *To make it easier,* decrease the reps, or don't lift as far off the floor. You can also substitute with bird dogs: position yourself on all fours on the floor and extend one arm out in front of you while also extending the opposite leg out behind you, keeping your weight centered; then switch the arm and leg.

DAY 25: KISS

You've got just six days left in the Core 4 program . . . hard to believe! You're rockin' it. Let's get right into today's topic because it's about magically freeing up more time in the day. I'm going to let you in on a secret way to find more time to get those things done that you never can seem to accomplish.

Ready?

It's called: Stop doing crap that isn't important.

I know, the sarcasm is thick. But seriously, how many times have you created stuff for yourself to do to be "busy" so that you just couldn't find time for things that really needed to get done? It seems to be part of human nature. You know you need to finish a work project—so you can free up the time to stop working extra hours on it at home—but instead you decide to alphabetize your spice rack or de-lint your couch.

Not that organized spices or a de-linted couch are bad, but you need to ask yourself, "What's the priority here?" (Remember the Values Inventory Worksheet from the Pillar 4 chapter, pages 80–81!)

The quote "Stop the glorification of busy" really resonates with me. How many people do you know who fill their lives with meaningless stuff only to appear busy and important? I can think of at least a few, and I'm guilty of it from time to time.

My point is that if there's something you want to accomplish, stop lollygagging around with less important things. Learn to prioritize. Take action on the most high-priority items by not doing the ones with lower priority. Remember your values and what matters to you most.

And to that, I say, "KISS," or "keep it super simple."

How to KISS

Do you *need* to make a twenty-five-ingredient, five-course dinner on a Tuesday night or will grilled chicken, sweet potato, and some spinach suffice? Three ingredients. Done.

Do you *need* to do five or six long workouts a week or is three enough? Three is probably plenty as long as they're challenging.

Do you *need* to please everyone and ignore yourself? No. Constantly ignoring your own needs and happiness only makes you a more miserable and exhausted human to be around.

I think you see where I'm going. Simplify your life. Declutter, physically and mentally. Streamline. Look for ways to be more efficient, not less. It all comes down to less drain on your energy.

Day 25 Challenge: Try to KISS

Pick one thing you can simplify or place as a higher priority and do it. If you have a bottomless to-do list, focus only on what you intend to do *today*.

DAY 26: TECH BOUNDARIES

I love keeping things simple. But when it comes to technology, well, simple goes flying out the window. Like it or not, technology is here to stay. Tech has enriched our lives in some ways . . . and made it more difficult in others. Try to imagine your daily life without technology. Hard, right?

Will we ever live in a world that has *less* technology than we do today? Doubtful. But it's easy to succumb—unless we're vigilant—to mindless tech consumption thanks to our brains. Many types of tech and social media platforms are designed specifically to be easy to use. *Very easy to use.* In fact, so easy to use you don't even think about it.

How? They help you complete the anticipation-reward loop I mentioned in the Pillar 3 chapter. The reward, you may think, will be a deeper or more convenient connection with people across the world or the ease of accomplishing tasks . . . but when you take a closer look, dopamine is at play.

Every hit of dopamine that comes with a ding from a new email or a text popping up is a reward. The problem is that dopamine's effect doesn't last. It's fleeting. So you end up needing more, seeking it out via technology, checking, scrolling, and refreshing, often mindlessly. It may all sound a little sinister, but tech companies *know* how your brain functions . . . and they leverage that to keep you using their platforms.

Think of social media and other forms of technology like junk food. It's delicious—so utterly delicious—because it pings all the right parts of your brain. But on a nutritional level, it sucks.

If tech is junk food, real-life relationships and interactions are like meat and veggies. Nourishing yourself with a base of meat and veggies, then eating junk food now and then, may be okay. Eating junk food 24/7 with the occasional meat and veggies tossed in? Not so much.

Creating Boundaries

Do you already have some boundaries about how you use technology? You may. But maybe it's time for some reflection.

I'm not suggesting you stop using all technology. But take a look at how much you use it, how it's making your life better (or not), and whether it's time to add more meat and veggies (in-person, real interaction) into your "diet."

For example, let's say you got into the not-so-great habit of lying in bed while checking social media on your phone. Not only does it send mixed messages about what the bed is actually for (sleeping and sex), you're plugged into the matrix until the very second you go to sleep.

Setting a boundary by charging your phone in the living room and plugging it in at least an hour before bedtime gives you a tech-free brain zone to help you decompress. Changing the habit may feel weird at first, but that's okay.

Another simple fix is turning off the incessant stream of notifications from your apps ("on" is usually their default setting). Or something more meaningful, like calling your loved ones instead of texting them.

It's up to you, but find at least one way today to feed yourself with the equivalent of meat and veggies instead of bingeing on tech "junk food."

Day 26 Challenge: Set One Tech Boundary, plus Work Out

Movements from last week make a dynamic warm-up. Complete all sets and reps of each movement before moving on to the next.

LEVEL 1

SUMO DEADLIFTS—*4 sets of 12 reps*

Stand with your feet about six to eight inches outside your hips and hold dumbbells or a kettlebell in front of your thighs with an overhand grip. Engage your core and keep your neck neutral as you hinge forward, bend your knees, and lower the weights until they touch the floor. Remember to push the floor away with your legs instead of lifting with your back. Return to the starting position, keeping the weight close to your body.

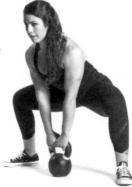
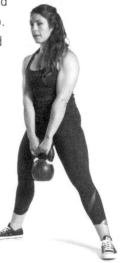

ALTERNATING LUNGES—*3 sets of 12 reps with each leg*

Stand with your feet under your hips, holding dumbbells in both hands. Step forward and bend your right knee to make a 90-degree angle with your right leg as you lower your left knee toward the floor. Drive through your front foot. Step forward with your left leg to bring your feet together. Repeat the movements on the opposite leg.

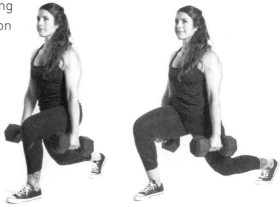

Pro Tips

» Make your step short enough that you can return to standing without swinging your torso.

» *To make it harder,* make them walking lunges, or hold the dumbbells over your head while you lunge.

ALTERNATING DUMBBELL SHOULDER PRESSES—*3 sets of 10 reps with each arm*

Stand with your feet under your hips and with dumbbells in both hands held at shoulder height, with your knuckles facing your shoulders. Engage your core, squeeze your butt, and keep your neck neutral as you actively push up through the shoulder to raise one dumbbell toward the ceiling. Keep your arm close to your head. Also, pull your ribs down instead of flaring them out. Lower the dumbbell and repeat the movements with the opposite arm.

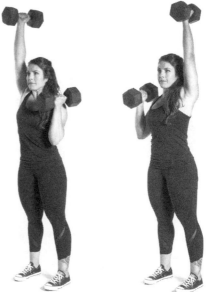

Pro Tip

» *To make it harder,* press both dumbbells up at the same time, or use a barbell.

SKULL CRUSHERS—*3 sets of 10 reps*

Lie on a weight bench, or on the floor with your knees bent and your feet flat on the floor, and hold one end of a dumbbell in your hands as pictured, with your arms extended. Engage your core as you bend your elbows to lower the dumbbell straight down toward the top of your head. Pull your ribs down instead of flaring them out. Then straighten your arms again, focusing on the triceps—the backs of the upper arms—to return the dumbbell to the starting position.

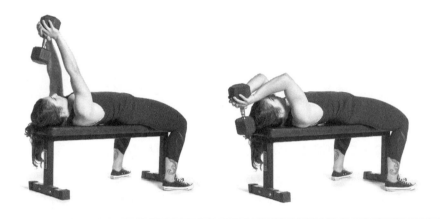

PULL-UPS—*4 sets of 6 to 8 reps*

Stand under a pull-up bar with your hands gripping the bar underhand or overhand (your choice) and shoulder width apart. Your thumbs should be wrapped all the way around the bar. Inhale as you engage your core and pull your body up until your chin clears the bar. Keep your neck neutral—don't crane your chin over the bar. Then lower back to the starting position with control to protect your shoulders.

Pro Tips

» *To make it easier,* secure a band around the bar and place your feet in it to reduce the amount of weight you're pulling up. Or start at the top of the pull-up position and then lower yourself down instead of doing the complete rep.

PLANKS—*4 sets of 30 to 45 seconds*

Lie on the floor facedown with your hands next to your chest and your elbows close to your sides. Take a breath and push your body up onto your toes and hands, engaging your core and keeping your body in a straight line. Don't stick your butt up in the air or let your hips sag. Hold this position, breathing normally.

Pro Tip

» *To make it harder,* add weight to your back, or lift one leg off the floor.

LEVEL 2

BARBELL BACK SQUATS—*3 sets of 3 reps at RPE 7*

Stand with a barbell resting across the meaty back of your shoulders, called the trapezius muscles, and held in an overhand grip. Don't let the barbell rest on your neck bones. Inhale, engage your core, squeeze your glutes, and hinge at the hip before bending your knees to lower your butt toward the floor until your thighs are parallel to the floor or slightly lower. Keep your neck neutral and your chest high, then return to the starting position, exhaling on the way up.

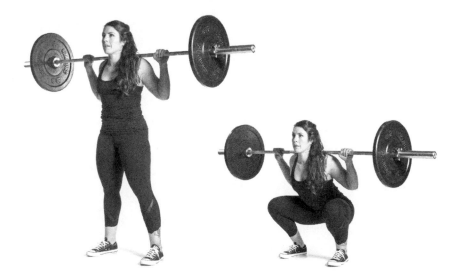

BARBELL SHOULDER PRESSES—*3 sets of 3 reps at RPE 7*

Stand with your feet under your hips and holding a barbell across the front of your shoulders with an overhand grip. Your hands should be slightly wider than shoulder width apart. Engage your core and press the barbell toward the ceiling. Maintain a neutral posture and pull your ribs down instead of flaring them out. Return to the starting position.

PULL-UPS—*4 sets of 5 or more reps*

Stand under a pull-up bar with your hands gripping the bar underhand or overhand (your choice) and shoulder width apart. Your thumbs should be wrapped all the way around the bar. Inhale as you engage your core and pull your body up until your chin clears the bar. Keep your neck neutral—don't crane your chin over the bar. Then lower back to the starting position with control to protect your shoulders.

Pro Tips

» *To make it easier,* secure a band around the bar and place your feet in it to reduce the amount of weight you're pulling up. Or start at the top of the pull-up position and then lower yourself down instead of doing the complete rep.

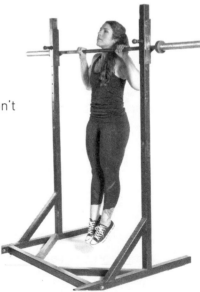

PLANKS—*4 sets of 30 to 45 seconds*

Lie on the floor facedown with your hands next to your chest and your elbows close to your sides. Take a breath and push your body up onto your toes and hands, engaging your core and keeping your body in a straight line. Don't stick your butt up in the air or let your hips sag. Hold this position, breathing normally.

Pro Tip

» *To make it harder*, add weight to your back, or lift one leg off the floor.

DAY 27: YOUR CIRCLE

Yesterday you learned that there is no substitute for the real-life connections you have. Today you'll focus on the special people in your life.

When I was a triathlete, my weakest discipline was swimming. I was a back-of-the-pack swimmer, but no matter how much I struggled, I always reminded myself to just keep moving forward, even if it meant doing the dog paddle or backstroke (which, incidentally, I had to do a lot).

Whenever you make big changes or try new things, it can be really scary. (Remember what you learned about fear on Day 18?) You may feel tons of uncertainty, but the most important thing to do is to move forward even if you're taking baby steps. Taking action when you're afraid is better than letting fear stop you cold.

Even the strongest, most self-directed people need support from time to time. You may be all Ms. Independent, saying, "I don't *need* anyone. I can do it myself." But chances are there's someone somewhere who has supported, guided, cheered, or motivated you.

It's hard to do big courageous things completely in solitude. Not impossible, just less common than you'd think.

Your Circle

Who has stood by you?

Who has offered you a helping hand when you needed it?

Who has given a shoulder for you to lean on?

Who has kicked your butt and told you that you're not quitting?

Who has encouraged you to be your best?

Your answers to these questions may be all the same person or different people. Make a mental note of who they are.

Now think about who has given you grief, stood in your way, been a roadblock, told you that you can't, etc. Often we have people in our lives who do nothing but tear us down. If you're a loyal person, you may find it difficult to step away from the people in your life who are blocking you.

Weeding the Friend Garden

If there's someone in your life who keeps crapping on your dreams, you don't have to stay friends. You *can* set boundaries. Step into your inner power and take responsibility.

Relationships are tricky, and sometimes they run their course. It's worth reflecting on. If someone's holding you back, what are you going to do about it?

You have a choice: either weed the friend garden or continue letting others keep you down. But you know the latter isn't what strong women do. If a friendship is not serving you anymore, wish the person well and move on.

Day 27 Challenge: Call, Write, or Talk to Three People Who Have Supported You When You Needed It Most

A simple "Thank you for being there for me" could be the highlight of their day. Of course, you can make it more in-depth. Cultivating an attitude of gratitude is one of the best ways to feel high on life. It works. Try it.

OPTIONAL WEEKEND WORKOUT. Do 4 rounds of the following exercises, resting 2 minutes after each round.

PULL-UPS (OR ALTERNATING DUMBBELL ROWS, PAGE 221)—4

Stand under a pull-up bar with your hands gripping the bar underhand or overhand (your choice) and shoulder width apart. Your thumbs should be wrapped all the way around the bar. Inhale as you engage your core and pull your body up until your chin clears the bar. Keep your neck neutral—don't crane your chin over the bar. Then lower back to the starting position with control to protect your shoulders.

Pro Tips

» *To make it easier,* secure a band around the bar and place your feet in it to reduce the amount of weight you're pulling up. Or start at the top of the pull-up position and then lower yourself down instead of doing the complete rep.

RENEGADE ROWS—*6 on each arm*

Lie facedown on the floor with dumbbells on either side of your body at about chest level. While grasping the dumbbells, push your body up into a plank position. Shift your weight onto your right arm and bend your left arm to row that dumbbell up to the left side of your rib cage. Actively pull with the upper back into each row, keeping the arm close to your body. Lower the dumbbell to the floor and repeat the movements with the other arm.

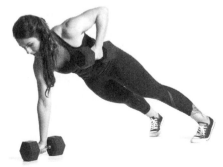

WALKING LUNGES—*8 with each leg*

Stand with your feet under your hips, holding dumbbells in both hands. Step forward and bend your right knee to make a 90-degree angle with your right leg as you lower your left knee toward the floor. Drive through your front foot. Step forward with your left leg and repeat the movements on the opposite leg, walking slowly forward.

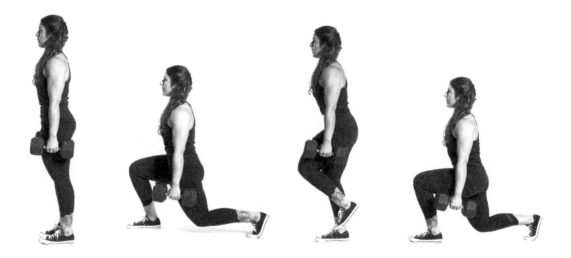

Pro Tip

» *To make it harder,* hold the dumbbells over your head while you lunge.

DAY 28: GRATITUDE

Yesterday's challenge may have left you feeling a little warm and fuzzy inside. You know what? That's a good thing. Let's keep that going today. There's one simple practice that can make an enormous impact on your life. It's so simple that it seems too good to be true. It's gratitude.

Gratitude is defined as "the quality of being thankful." Today's stressful modern world often magnifies what we're lacking and distracts us from taking the time to

express our thankfulness. There's compelling research from Dr. Robert Emmons of UC Davis demonstrating the positive effects of practicing gratitude, including

better, more restful sleep;

lower blood pressure;

stronger immunity;

greater happiness;

deeper feelings of social confidence; and

more compassion for others.

It appears that the benefits of practicing gratitude come directly from a decrease in stress. Simply put, when you're grateful, it's easier to stay grounded in the present (instead of feeling stressed about the past or the future). This brings positive emotions to the forefront. Staying aware of the good you have in your life means you focus less on the bad.

There's an interesting paradox about happiness that's also been studied by scientists: happiness is both a cause and an effect of success. Most people treat happiness as an effect: "I'll be happy when I lose those last 10 pounds." "I'll feel better about myself when I get that raise." "Life will be happy when I find the perfect mate."

But the most successful people—the ones who meet their goals—know that they must *cultivate* happiness in order to find success. Happiness and other positive emotions expand your thinking and creativity, quite the opposite of what occurs when you're stressed. Stress makes it harder to see alternative solutions to your problems. By including gratitude as a practice, you bolster positive emotions and happiness, which are a cause of success as much as they are an effect.

Practice Makes Perfect

The great lie perpetuated by our technology-driven world—where we voyeuristically peek into other people's lives—is that, gosh darn it, they're so much happier than we are. It seems others are blessed with big, fun, exciting things and, well, we lead bland lives by comparison.

Remember that what you see on social media and TV is a filtered, curated view. People less frequently share their struggles and dark times or even the mundane but satisfying moments.

The antidote is developing a keen eye for small but joyful moments that pop up in your everyday life. The big, fun, exciting things may happen only once in a blue moon. The little, joyful things happen all the time . . . even when you're going through a rough patch. There's always sunlight.

But much like you can't build muscle by just staring at a dumbbell, you can't develop more happiness and enjoy the benefits of gratitude without practice. One place to start is simply by noticing such things. When something heartwarming, joyful, and gratifying happens, it's time to take note.

A mental note is great—sit in that moment and savor it—but writing it down is even more powerful. My favorite personal practice, and one that's helped my clients immensely, is keeping a gratitude journal. The secret is to get detailed about what you're thankful for. And, of course, writing in the journal on a regular basis. Keep it by your bedside and jot down a few things you were grateful for that day.

Instead of saying "I'm thankful for my husband," I might say "I'm thankful my husband got up early and made me a cup of coffee in my favorite mug." Be really specific—the more detailed, the better. Noticing distinct moments instead of just using blanket statements will help you hone your eye and heart—for moments of gratitude.

Day 28 Challenge: Start a Daily Practice of Writing Down What You're Grateful for, plus Work Out

I recommend writing in your gratitude journal at night before bed, but there's no wrong way to do it. Start with three to five things you're grateful for, and remember to give special attention to the small and even "mundane" things.

As far as the workout, movements from last week make a dynamic warm-up. Complete all sets and reps of each movement before moving on to the next.

LEVEL 1

GLUTE BRIDGES—*4 sets of 12 reps*

Lie on your back with your knees bent, your feet flat on the floor and close to your hips, and your arms at your sides on the floor. Engage your core and squeeze your butt as you slowly drive your hips up toward the ceiling so that your body is in a straight line from head to knees. Keep your knees parallel to each other; don't let them collapse in or out. Slowly lower your hips back to the starting position.

Pro Tip

» *To make it harder,* lift up one leg at a time from the bridge position.

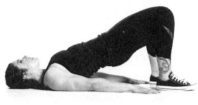

WALKING LUNGES—*4 sets of 10 reps with each leg*

Stand with your feet under your hips, holding dumbbells in both hands. Step forward and bend your right knee to make a 90-degree angle with your right leg as you lower your left knee toward the floor. Drive through the heel of your front foot as you step forward with your left leg and repeat the movements on the opposite leg, walking slowly forward.

Pro Tip

» *To make it harder,* hold the dumbbells over your head while you lunge.

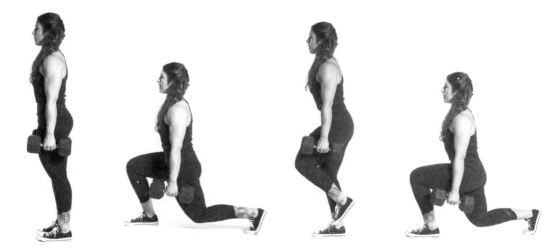

ALTERNATING DUMBBELL SHOULDER PRESSES—*3 sets of 10 reps with each arm*

Stand with your feet under your hips and with dumbbells in both hands held at shoulder height, with your knuckles facing your shoulders. Engage your core, squeeze your butt, and keep your neck neutral as you actively push up through the shoulder to raise one dumbbell toward the ceiling. Keep your arm close to your head. Also, pull your ribs down instead of flaring them out. Lower the dumbbell and repeat the movements with the opposite arm.

Pro Tip

» *To make it harder,* press both dumbbells up at the same time or use a barbell.

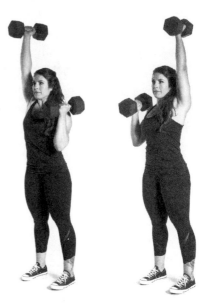

ALTERNATING DUMBBELL ROWS—*4 sets of 8 reps with each arm*

Holding a dumbbell in your left hand, to begin with, stand with your right foot forward in a partial lunge and your body from your left heel to the top of your head forming almost a straight line. Keep your abs engaged, your spine aligned, and your elbow close to your body as you pull the dumbbell up to your ribs, then lower it. You can rest your other hand on your knee or your leg for support. Repeat the movements on the opposite side.

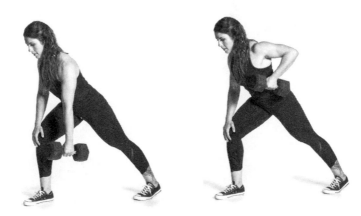

MOUNTAIN CLIMBERS—*3 sets of 12 reps with each leg*

Get on the floor in the plank position, with your hands shoulder width apart. Engage your core as you quickly pull one knee toward your chest, just touching your foot to the floor before extending that leg back again. Repeat the movement with the opposite leg. Continue to alternate legs.

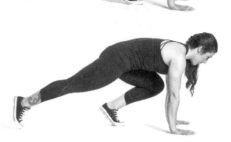

Pro Tip

» *To make it harder,* increase the pace.

LEVEL 2

BARBELL BACK SQUATS—*3 sets of 2 at RPE 8*

Stand with a barbell resting across the meaty back of your shoulders, called the trapezius muscles, and held in an overhand grip. Don't let the barbell rest on your neck bones. Inhale, engage your core, squeeze your glutes, and hinge at the hip before bending your knees to lower your butt toward the floor until your thighs are parallel to the floor or slightly lower. Keep your neck neutral and your chest high, then return to the starting position, exhaling on the way up.

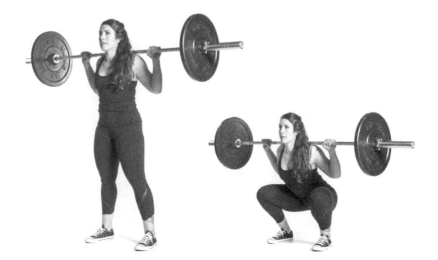

BARBELL POWER CLEANS—*up to 3 sets of 1 rep at RPE 7+*

Stand with your feet slightly wider than hip width apart and with a barbell on the floor in front of your feet. Hinge at the hips and grab the barbell overhand with your hands positioned just outside your hips. Lift it to your thighs, then push with your legs and jump as you bend your elbows to flip the bar up and shrug it to your shoulders. The power comes from your legs driving the bar up rather than pulling it with your arms. Stand in a partial squat with your knees slightly bent. Pause briefly, then return the bar to the floor.

Pro Tip

» *To make it harder,* use an unbalanced object like a sandbag, or receive the weight in a full squat clean.

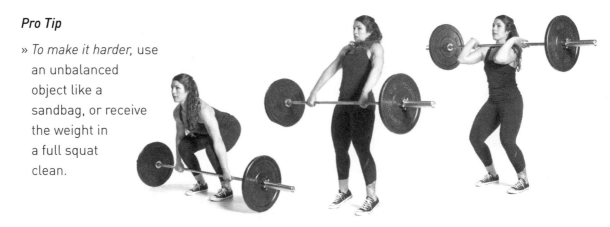

PUSH-UPS—*4 sets of the maximum reps you can do*

Lie facedown on the floor and place your hands on the floor next to your body at about chest level, with your elbows close to your sides. Your body should look like an arrow if you could view it from above, not the letter T. Push your body up so that you're on your hands and toes, keeping your body in a straight line. Don't stick your butt up into the air or drop your butt too low. Bend your elbows to lower your chest toward the floor, and then push back up. As you push up, take a breath and keep your butt and core tight.

Pro Tip

» *To make it harder,* add weight on your back, or try clapping push-ups.

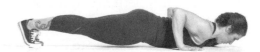

HOLLOW ROCKS—*4 sets of 10 to 15 reps*

Lie on your back with your arms extended above your head. Engage your core and raise your legs and arms at the same time, pointing your toes and keeping your arms close to your ears. Press your lower back to the floor as you rock lightly back and forth, maintaining the same body position and breathing normally. Relax down into your starting position.

Pro Tip

» *To make it harder,* hang by your arms from a pull-up bar instead, squeeze your butt, brace your core, and pull your knees up toward your elbows, crunching your abs.

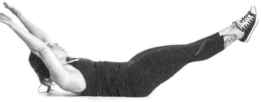

DAY 29: PURPOSE

Today we'll pull back a bit to take a 30,000-foot view and talk about a big picture topic: purpose.

Some people associate purpose with living to a higher potential or to serve others in the world. When there's misalignment between your purpose and what you actually do in the world, you're likely to feel a drain on your energy. Sometimes it shows up as a lack of fulfillment with career. Other times, it's a feeling of drifting aimlessly like a ship without a sail.

Perhaps one of the simplest ways to look at purpose is inspired by author Tony Schwartz. He succinctly defines purpose as what happens when your values meet your actions. A clear sense of purpose results when the two align. A lack of purpose results when they don't.

Remember your Values Inventory Worksheet (pages 80–81) in the Pillar 4 chapter? Your values are what you hold to be true in life, the guiding principles you live by, and the things that are important to you. Some values are intrinsic, such as creativity and honesty. Some are extrinsic, like the need for recognition or status. And one type isn't inherently better than the other, but most people find intrinsic values to be more satisfying and less fleeting. When what you do in the world—your actions—matches your values, you're likely to feel a clear sense of purpose.

How to Look Outside Yourself

In the Core 4 program, you've done a lot of work on your internal landscape. Taking care of yourself and attending to your basic needs is very important. And in times of extra stress, I highly recommend my clients prioritize this kind of self-care. It's not to be selfish or ignore your other responsibilities. Rather, it's because you'll have extra energy, patience, and joy when caring for others if you've taken care of yourself first.

When you're more relaxed, your metaphorical blinders are taken off. Your perspective widens and you see solutions where previously there appeared to be none. When you're stressed, however, you're in blinders mode. Everything narrows. Time slips away too fast. That's when it's time to buckle down and take care of you.

Once you start filling your cup again, you're better able to care for others.

Please don't mistake what I'm saying. Serving others with energy you do not have is not sustainable. That would be like feeding the poor by maxing out your credit card. You're spending money you don't have, and it's going to catch up with you in the end.

Instead, what if you round up on every debit card purchase you make for a year and put that money into a special account . . . then you donate what you've saved up? Think about building up enough extra energy so you can give of that surplus freely to others without dipping into your own "account."

Service to others is one of the most fulfilling ways to connect with your purpose, but putting your health and wellness in jeopardy to do it might not be worth it in the end. Take care of you, then give to others to bolster your sense of purpose and community in ways that align with your values.

Day 29 Challenge: Complete the Values Inventory Worksheet

If you haven't already, fill out the Values Inventory Worksheet and give some thought to what you came up with (pages 80–81).

DAY 30: BUILD LASTING HABITS

Welcome to the last day! You learned on Day 28 that getting grateful is a powerful way to focus your attention on all the good stuff you've got in your life. Do it often enough and it becomes a habit. But what about your not-so-awesome habits?

All you have to do is type "break a habit" into Google, and you'll get a staggering 46 million plus hits. The term "break a bad habit" has been repeated so much it's practically fact. But is it?

In *The Power of Habit*, Charles Duhigg presents an incredibly useful way of understanding habits: they can't be broken, but they can be worked around. Duhigg explains that once a habit develops, it's there to stay, because you've created neural pathways in your brain that automate the behavior.

To deal with a habit you don't want anymore, *create a new habit* in its place that will override the old one.

My client Melissa had a habit of drinking wine after dinner. At a certain point she decided it was time to take a break from wine. It was disrupting her sleep, and the empty calories each night weren't helping her body composition goals.

Instead of just telling Melissa to stop drinking wine—which would likely result in a battle of willpower—we worked together to create a different habit that could take its place. She started off thinking she needed to drink something else to keep her hands busy. When I asked her to get clear about *why* she drank the wine, it wasn't because she was hungry or thirsty or bored. It was to deal with the stress of the day. So Melissa came up with a new habit that worked better: writing in her journal.

There's also no set amount of time it takes to create or replace a habit in the first place. It differs from person to person and habit to habit. The oft-repeated statement "It takes twenty-one days to form a new habit" is not supported by what happens in the real world. Sometimes it's faster, sometimes slower.

Looking Deeper into Habits

To really understand your habits, it helps to look deeper and consider these questions:

Are there any cues that cause you to repeat the habit? For Melissa, it was the time of day—after dinner.

What do you get from repeating the habit? Does it provide escape from something boring or painful? Maybe it's stimulating, providing energy or connection with another person. Melissa hypothesized that wine rewarded her with an escape from stress. She replaced her wine habit with a bath and journaling after dinner to cope with the stress of her day . . . and it became a lasting replacement for her glass of merlot.

To effectively build new habits in place of the old ones, you have to drill down to figure out what the reward is. And just because a new behavior seems promising on paper doesn't mean it will stick when you try it out in the real world. That's why you sometimes have to try again until you find a better behavior that sticks around until it becomes more automatic.

Day 30 Challenge: Journal About a Habit You Currently Have That You'd Like to Replace, plus Work Out

Identify the cues and benefits of a habit you'd like to change. Brainstorm a few new behaviors you could substitute for the old one. Over the course of the next week or two, try implementing the new behaviors. If something doesn't stick, try again!

As always with this workout, the movements from last week make a dynamic warm-up. Complete all sets and reps of each movement before moving on to the next.

TURKISH GET-UPS—*1 set of 5 reps on each side*

Lie on the floor holding a dumbbell or kettlebell in your right hand, with your arm pointed straight up at the ceiling. Keep your eyes on the weight above you as you bend your right knee to bring your right foot flat onto the floor next to your hip. Engage your core as you press up onto your left elbow, then your left hand. Slide your left leg back between your left arm and right foot so that you're kneeling on your left knee, then lift your left hand off the floor. Go slowly and find stability in each position. Continue to keep your eyes on the weight as you return to the starting position by reversing your movements.

Pro Tips

» *To make it easier,* do all the moves without a weight.

» *To make it harder,* after you lift your hand from the floor, fully stand up while again continuing to keep your eyes on the weight above you.

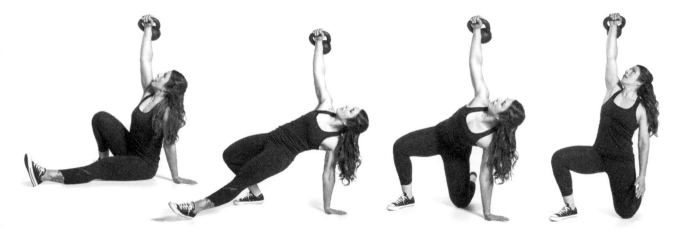

GOBLET SQUATS—*4 sets of 12 reps*

Stand with your feet slightly wider than hip width and hold a dumbbell or kettlebell in front of your chest. Inhale and engage your core as you hinge from your hips and bend your knees to lower your bottom toward the floor, keeping your feet in a comfortable squat stance with your thighs a little lower than parallel. Exhale as you return to the starting position.

SPLIT SQUATS—*4 sets of 10 reps with each leg*

Stand with your feet under your hips and with dumbbells held at shoulder height. Step forward with your left leg into a lunge stance. Engage your core and gently lower your right knee toward the floor. Return to a standing position, then lower your right knee again. Do all reps on this leg before driving through your front foot, engaging your glutes, and returning to the starting position. Repeat with opposite leg positions.

Pro Tip

» *To make it harder,* place your back foot up on a bench (to do a Bulgarian split squat).

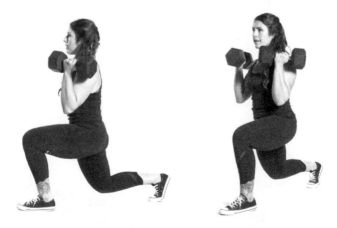

PUSH-UPS—*3 sets of 10 reps*

Lie facedown on the floor and place your hands on the floor next to your body at about chest level, with your elbows close to your sides. Your body should look like an arrow if you could view it from above, not the letter T. Push your body up so that you're on your hands and toes, keeping your body in a straight line. Don't stick your butt up into the air or drop your butt too low. Bend your elbows to lower your chest toward the floor, and then push back up. As you push up, take a breath and keep your butt and core tight.

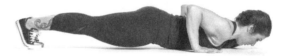

Pro Tip

» *To make it harder,* add weight on your back, or try clapping push-ups.

HOLLOW ROCKS—*4 sets of 10 to 15 reps*

Lie on your back with your arms extended above your head. Engage your core and raise your legs and arms at the same time, pointing your toes and keeping your arms close to your ears. Press your lower back to the floor as you rock lightly back and forth, maintaining the same body position and breathing normally. Relax down into your starting position.

Pro Tip

» *To make it harder,* hang by your arms from a pull-up bar instead, squeeze your butt, brace your core, and pull your knees up toward your elbows, crunching your abs.

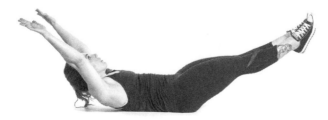

LEVEL 2

BARBELL DEADLIFTS—*1 set of 3 reps at RPE 8*

Stand with your feet under your hips with a barbell on the floor close to your shins. Hinge at the hips and grasp the barbell overhand with your hands positioned just outside your hips. Inhale, engage your core, squeeze your glutes, and push the floor away with your legs instead of lifting your back to raise the barbell. Keep your neck neutral and the barbell close to your body as you come to a standing position, exhaling on the way up. Be sure to keep your toes from lifting off the floor throughout the movement. Hinge forward at the hips, lower the weight to the floor, and return to the starting position.

BARBELL SHOULDER PRESSES—*3 sets of 5 reps at RPE 7*

Stand with your feet under your hips and holding a barbell across the front of your shoulders with an overhand grip. Your hands should be slightly wider than shoulder width apart. Engage your core and press the barbell toward the ceiling. Maintain a neutral posture and pull your ribs down instead of flaring them out. Return to the starting position.

PULL-UPS—*4 sets of 5 or more reps*

Stand under a pull-up bar with your hands gripping the bar underhand or overhand (your choice) and shoulder width apart. Your thumbs should be wrapped all the way around the bar. Inhale as you engage your core and pull your body up until your chin clears the bar. Keep your neck neutral—don't crane your chin over the bar. Then lower back to the starting position with control to protect your shoulders.

Pro Tips

» *To make it easier,* secure a band around the bar and place your feet in it to reduce the amount of weight you're pulling up. Or start at the top of the pull-up position and then lower yourself down instead of doing the complete rep.

TURKISH GET-UPS—*1 set of 5 reps on each side*

Lie on the floor holding a dumbbell or kettlebell in your right hand, with your arm pointed straight up at the ceiling. Keep your eyes on the weight above you as you bend your right knee to bring your right foot flat onto the floor next to your hip. Engage your core as you press up onto your left elbow, then your left hand. Slide your left leg back between your left arm and right foot so that you're kneeling on your left knee, then lift your left hand off the floor. Continue to keep your eyes on the weight above you as you fully stand up. Go slowly and find stability in each position. Then return to the starting position by reversing your movements.

Pro Tip

» *To make it easier,* do all the moves without a weight, or practice the first half of the movements without involving the legs.

CONCLUSION

Day 31

You did it! You rocked the Core 4 program! And you may be thinking, *So, what's next?*

That's up to you. The whole point of the Core 4 framework is to give you a fun structure for trying out lots of new tools and techniques to improve your health and happiness. I don't recommend doing it over and over forever like a continuous loop. Eventually you've got to go live your life and do the best you can with what you've got at any given time. Plus, life is guaranteed to change, so what works for you now may not work for you in six months, a year, or ten years. In other words, stay adaptable and commit to growth if you want to take up more space and get stronger.

You've tested a slew of powerful tools and added them to your health toolbox, and you can pull them out as you need to. One of the most effective is your Personal Pillar Plan (pages 84–85). Use it as a guide, coming back to it and adjusting when necessary. That will help you break from drifting aimlessly or avoiding areas where you know you could improve.

Another helpful tool is the Health Tracker you filled out in the "Get Ready" chapter before the Core 4 program began. Revisit that questionnaire now (pages 102–103). Then return and answer the following questions:

Consider your Day 1 answers and compare them to how you answered today, on Day 31. What has improved?

Did anything not improve? If so, what, and why do you think that is?

Make some general conclusions about how your health has changed in the last 30 days. How have you strengthened your Core 4?

DOING THE CORE 4 PROGRAM AGAIN

When you feel discomfort, I don't want you to run back to the program. Instead, I want you to open your metaphorical toolbox and apply one of the tools you've learned from this book to your life. You may have learned things in the Core 4 that aren't really relevant to you at this point. But having access to them may help you down the road.

You *will* continue to change. As soon as you get comfortable, life may throw you for a loop. The point isn't to start another 30-day program to "get control" but rather to dip back into the tools when you need them. Maybe you're feeling overwhelmed at the idea of relocating or taking a new job or even starting a new relationship, and you think, *Hey, there was a challenge about fear. I'm going to go back and read through that day again.*

The point is progress, not perfection. You've got this framework to help you navigate your way, along with your intuition. You won't be roaming around the internet collecting conflicting information and getting overwhelmed with next steps. You can choose how to make the strategies and the Core 4 pillars work for your life and what matters to you.

As I said in the introduction, this program is designed to give you both boundaries and freedom—a framework, if you will. No longer are you at the edge of a deep, dark forest with no navigational tools and no path. You're prepared! What do I hope for you? To grow and expand beyond the experience of this book the way Gina, age forty-six, has, as she explained a year after doing the Core 4 program:

There are no hard-set "rules" you have to follow or you're going to be a failure. This program is a gentle teacher helping people figure out their own path to overall health (mind, body, and spirit). And it's a windy, curvy path that each person has to take on their own. What's important to one person won't be as important to another . . .

I also like that this is a lifelong process, so we have access to it forever. I'm continually working on different aspects, or I'll go back and redo a lesson. I've mainly focused on the mindset and energy pillars for the past year, but that has helped me heal enough that I'm now ready to revisit the strength and food pillars. If I'd tried to focus on those in the beginning, I really believe I wouldn't have kept with the program. It would have been too much like a "diet." I appreciate Steph's outlook and "tough love" when needed. It's always grounded in reality, and it's helped many people regain their own inner power.

Finding that kind of power is what can launch you into the life you've dreamed of living. Michelle, age twenty-six, started Core 4 with a focus on changing her body:

I had been aimlessly going to the gym with the mindset of "I just want to lose weight" and would frequently hit up the elliptical and treadmill and sometimes used the weight lifting machines. I had no clue what I was doing, and I was there for all the wrong reasons. I wanted to learn about how to properly strengthen my body, how to properly do various exercises, and still I wanted to "tone" and lose weight. Additionally, I was interested in curbing my bad eating habits, which included overindulging, snacking excessively, and eating foods that were making me feel bad.

Her results far exceeded her initial hopes and goals.

Not to be overdramatic, but I gained the world with this challenge. I went in wanting to focus on eating nourishing foods and strengthening my body but ended up almost exclusively focusing on recharging my energy and mastering my mindset. Before this challenge I didn't think those two pillars were my problem, but through this challenge I learned that they were my biggest problems to achieving a happier, healthier, and harder-to-kill me. This challenge challenged me to really consider how I was talking to myself, how I was presenting myself to the world, how tired I was, and how ready I was to give myself what I deserved. This challenge gave me more confidence in myself and it gave me strength to make some tough decisions.

I learned how to properly recharge, which seriously made the biggest difference in my day-to-day life. This challenge helped me to focus on areas that are traditionally

left out of health and fitness programs, which in turn helped me to gain strength, make better eating decisions, and develop good habits. Additionally, by addressing the Recharge Your Energy and Empower Your Mind pillars I was able to make life-changing decisions that, one year later, have landed me in my dream job and exactly where I want to be in life right now.

To live your best life—most goals boil down to this, right? When you reconnect with your inner power and listen to your inner voice, you'll be able to get there. And if you feel discouraged, remember that it's normal to experience progress and then setbacks, progress and setbacks. You're not going to rocket off into the future without any stumbles. Part of the learning process is making mistakes—getting stuck and having to figure your way out of it. It's when you push through a sticking point that you get to a new level of understanding.

If you slip back into your old habits, now you have self-awareness. You have tools you didn't have before. You know how to create new routines. Now you can look at it not as a failure but as a minor setback. You will use that setback as a platform for going forward. It's a speed bump—it may slow you, but it won't stop you.

You've learned to listen to your inner voice. You've tapped into your own power—power that you may have forgotten you had, but you've embraced it now. You're not the same person you were before you started the Core 4 program. Now get out there and live your biggest, boldest, fiercest life.

The Core 4 Recipes

Eating nourishing food shouldn't be complicated. I've put together thirty diverse recipes you can enjoy as part of the Core 4 meal plan or as stand-alone inspiration. Remember to have fun with them: cooking isn't as precise as baking, and you can usually swap in a similar herb, spice, vegetable, or meat if you don't have something on hand. But remember to include the nourishing foods in the Pillar 1 chapter (see the Nourishing Foods Framework, pages 34–35).

Feeling a little freaked out? It's okay. Deep breath. It may be weird AF at first, but just like anything else, a little practice goes a long way.

All the recipes in the Core 4 are gluten-free. Some mention the optional add of dairy, legumes, nuts, or the occasional natural sweetener. If there are foods you are sensitive or allergic to, you can make a substitution and it'll still be delish. Often I've offered a choice between ingredients, like olive oil or ghee, for example. Or I've listed an ingredient like cheese as "optional." When that's the case, the recipe is still labeled "dairy-free" because you have the option to make it so. And I've included lots of ideas for changing it up to suit your needs, such as carb-ing a dish up or down and alternative cooking methods.

Let's dig in!

QUICK SIDE DISHES

ROASTED POTATOES AND SWEET POTATOES: Preheat the oven to 400°F. Place whole, unpeeled potatoes or sweet potatoes on a parchment-lined baking sheet and roast them for 45 to 60 minutes or until they're tender when pierced with a fork.

ROASTED VEGGIES: Preheat the oven to 400°F. Chop up your choice of veggies and toss them in olive oil or melted ghee, salt, and pepper. Roast the veggies on a parchment-lined baking sheet for 20 to 40 minutes, or until they're tender when pierced with a fork and golden around the edges. Make sure to stir them halfway through the roasting process for even cooking. Harder veggies will take longer to cook.

STEAMED GREENS: Wash, then chop your choice of greens. Set a steamer basket in a medium pot and add an inch or two of water to the pot. Set the pot over high heat, put the lid on, and bring the water to a boil. Add the greens to the steamer basket. Cover and steam them until they're lightly wilted, about 3 to 5 minutes. Season with salt and pepper before serving.

HARD-BOILED EGGS: I like steaming whole eggs for the easiest peeling ever, even when the eggs are fresh. Set a steamer basket in a medium pot and add an inch or two of water to the pot. Set the pot over high heat, put the lid on, and bring the water to a boil. Add the whole eggs to the steamer basket, and steam them for 8 minutes with the lid on. While the eggs are steaming, fill a medium to large bowl with ice and water. When the eggs are ready, plunge them into the ice water until they cool. Keep the shells on until you're ready to eat them.

BAKED CHICKEN: Preheat the oven to 425°F. Line a rimmed baking sheet or baking dish with parchment paper. Wash the chicken and pat it dry with paper towels. Place it on the baking sheet or dish and sprinkle it with salt and pepper. Roast it for 20 minutes, then reduce the heat to 300°F. Roast it for another 45 minutes or until the chicken is cooked through.

BAKED BACON: Preheat the oven to 350°F. Bake the bacon on a parchment-lined baking sheet for 10 to 20 minutes, depending on the thickness of the bacon and your desired crispiness. You may want to save the bacon fat in a jar for other cooking.

CHICKEN SAUSAGE: Cook or reheat the sausages according to the package directions, or brown them on all sides evenly in a skillet set over medium heat. It may take 10 to 15 minutes for them to cook through. If you can't find sausage made without preservatives or questionable ingredients, buy plain ground chicken and brown it seasoned with cinnamon, allspice, ginger, nutmeg, salt, and pepper for a breakfast-style sausage.

Breakfast Sausage Casserole

GRAIN-FREE, NUT-FREE, DAIRY-FREE

This one-pan breakfast has all my fave first-meal-of-the-day features: hash browns, savory sausage, and tasty eggs. It comes together quickly, fills you up, and tastes even better the next day. If you can't find bulk sausage, grab regular sausages from your local market and squeeze out the filling—chicken or pork sausages work just fine.

PREP TIME: 10 MINUTES
COOKING TIME: 30 MINUTES
SERVES 4

Olive oil or ghee for cooking
12 ounces bulk pork breakfast
   sausage
1 poblano pepper, stemmed,
   seeded, and chopped
1 large shallot, sliced
1 pound Yukon gold potatoes,
   shredded or spiralized
9 large eggs
¼ cup coconut or almond milk
½ teaspoon smoked paprika
Pinch each of sea salt and
   ground black pepper
4 ounces shredded full-fat
   cheddar cheese, optional

Preheat the oven to 375°F.

In a large cast-iron skillet set over medium-high heat, warm about 2 teaspoons olive oil or ghee. Add the sausage, breaking it apart with a wooden spoon, then add the poblano pepper and shallot. Sauté the mixture for 5 to 7 minutes, stirring often, until the meat is cooked through and the veggies are softened. Remove the skillet from heat and transfer the meat to a bowl. Wipe out the skillet with a paper towel.

Set the same skillet over medium heat, and warm about 1 tablespoon olive oil or ghee. Add the potatoes in a single layer and gently press them down. Cook them for about 3 to 4 minutes or until the potatoes begin to lightly brown. Flip them and cook them another 3 to 4 minutes, then turn off the heat.

While the potatoes are browning, get the eggs ready. In a large bowl beat together the eggs, coconut or almond milk, smoked paprika, and salt and pepper with a fork or a whisk.

Now put it all together. Add the sausage-veggie mixture to the skillet on top of the potatoes. Then pour the egg mixture over everything. Place the entire skillet into the oven and bake the casserole for about 15 minutes or until the eggs are set. Top it with the optional cheddar cheese as soon as it comes out of the oven. Slice and serve.

Change It Up

– Use sweet potato or butternut squash "noodles" (use a vegetable spiralizer to make these) instead of Yukon gold potatoes.

– No oven-safe skillet? Layer the ingredients in a greased 9 × 13-inch glass baking dish and bake as instructed.

Italian Frittata

GRAIN-FREE, NUT-FREE, DAIRY-FREE

As far as one-pan breakfasts go, frittatas are the ultimate. Cook up the filling ingredients, add eggs, and bake. They're satisfying and portable. I love making my frittatas in a cast-iron skillet for ultimate stovetop-to-oven ease. As long as your skillet is well seasoned, the frittata won't stick. I love the flavors in this recipe, but feel free to customize it with your favorite ingredients.

PREP TIME: 10 MINUTES
COOKING TIME: 30 MINUTES
SERVES 4 TO 6

12 large eggs
¼ cup coconut milk
3 ounces sun-dried tomatoes, chopped
2 teaspoons dried basil
½ teaspoon sea salt
¾ teaspoon ground black pepper
Olive oil or ghee for cooking
8 ounces Italian chicken sausage, removed from casings
1 small yellow onion, sliced
3 to 4 handfuls of fresh spinach
2 Roma tomatoes, sliced
2 ounces soft goat cheese, optional

Preheat the oven to 375°F.

In a large bowl, whisk the eggs, then stir in the coconut milk, sun-dried tomatoes, basil, salt, and pepper. Set the mixture aside.

In a large cast-iron skillet set over medium-high heat, warm about 1 tablespoon olive oil or ghee. Add the sausage meat, breaking it apart with a wooden spoon, and cook it for 5 to 7 minutes, stirring often, or until the meat is cooked through. Add the onion and spinach, and continue cooking for about another 5 minutes, or until the onion is translucent.

Pour the egg mixture into the hot skillet over the meat and veggies. Give everything a stir, turn off the heat, and arrange the sliced tomatoes and optional goat cheese on top. Place the entire skillet in the oven and bake the frittata for about 20 minutes, or until the eggs are set. Slice and serve.

Change It Up

– Top with fresh basil.

– No oven-safe skillet? Combine the ingredients in a greased 9 × 13-inch glass baking dish and bake as instructed.

Savory Ham and Egg Cups

GRAIN-FREE, NUT-FREE, DAIRY-FREE

Need a portable but protein-packed breakfast? Heck yes, please and thank you. These ham and egg cups are ridiculously easy and bake while you're getting ready to get out the door and on with your day. The idea is simple: make a cup in a muffin tin with a thin slice of ham, then fill it with an egg, and add your favorite toppings. No paper muffin liners needed!

PREP TIME: 10 MINUTES
COOKING TIME: 15 MINUTES
SERVES 4 TO 6

Olive oil or ghee for greasing
12 slices high-quality deli ham
¼ cup packed spinach leaves,
　chopped
12 large eggs
6 cherry tomatoes, halved
2 ounces shredded full-fat
　cheddar cheese, optional

Preheat the oven to 350°F.

Lightly oil the muffin tin, then lay a slice of ham in each cup, pushing it down lightly until it forms a cup. Add a little chopped spinach to the bottom of each ham cup, then crack an egg into each. Top each cup with a halved cherry tomato and a pinch of the cheddar cheese if using.

Bake the cups for 16 to 18 minutes, or until the whites and yolks are set. Serve hot or cold.

Change It Up

– The flavor variations here are endless. Instead of salsa, add a dollop of pesto.

– Make these ahead and reheat by popping them into a 350°F oven for 15 to 20 minutes. If you freeze the cups, reheat them in a 350°F oven for 25 to 30 minutes.

Banana Cinnamon No-Oatmeal

GRAIN-FREE, VEGETARIAN, DAIRY-FREE, NIGHTSHADE-FREE

Sometimes you just want a comforting bowl of warmth for breakfast, but if oats don't work well for you, it can be hard to fill the gap. Enter my Banana Cinnamon No-Oatmeal. It has a similar texture and flavor, plus it's chock-full of protein and healthy fats that will keep you satiated—without the crash of refined carb breakfasts. And it comes together in just minutes. Sometimes I serve this alongside a warm salad just to sneak in some extra greens.

PREP TIME: 5 MINUTES
COOKING TIME: 5 MINUTES
SERVES 4

8 large eggs
2 ripe bananas
1 cup almond milk
2 Medjool dates, pitted
2 teaspoons vanilla extract
2 teaspoons ground cinnamon
1 cup shredded unsweetened
  coconut
½ cup ground flaxseed
2 tablespoons chia seeds
2 tablespoons hemp hearts
Pinch of sea salt

In a blender or food processor, purée the eggs, bananas, almond milk, dates, vanilla, and cinnamon for 30 seconds, or until the mixture is smooth. Set the mixture aside.

In a medium saucepan, combine the coconut, flaxseed, chia seeds, hemp hearts, and salt, then pour the egg and banana mixture into the saucepan. Set the pan over medium heat and whisk the ingredients together. Keep whisking and gently heating until the mixture thickens, but without letting it boil. This usually takes 5 minutes or less. Serve hot.

The no-oatmeal will continue to thicken as it stands and when refrigerated. To reheat it, warm it in a small saucepan with a splash or two of additional almond milk. Stir the mixture until it's warmed through.

Change It Up

– Add 2 more dates if you like your no-oatmeal a bit sweeter.

– Swap out the almond milk for coconut or cashew milk.

PB and J Chia Breakfast Cups

GRAIN-FREE, DAIRY-FREE, NIGHTSHADE-FREE, VEGETARIAN, EGG-FREE

What can you say about peanut butter and jelly? It's a classic and comforting flavor combination that can make just about anyone nostalgic for simpler times. I took the flavors of PB and J and infused them into these little chia seed puddings. The good news is that my spin is low in sugar so these won't send your blood sugar skyrocketing first thing in the morning. They're easy to make ahead of time so you have something healthy and filling ready before you dash out the door. Add 2 tablespoons of your favorite collagen powder for a protein boost.

PREP TIME: 10 MINUTES
COOKING TIME: 10 MINUTES
SETTING TIME: 2 HOURS
SERVES 4

12 ounces frozen unsweetened strawberries
2 cups almond or coconut milk
¼ cup unsweetened smooth peanut butter
1 tablespoon honey or maple syrup, optional
2 tablespoons collagen powder, optional
5 tablespoons chia seeds
2 tablespoons chopped peanuts or almonds for garnish, optional
Fresh strawberries for garnish, optional

In a small saucepan set over medium-low heat, cook the frozen strawberries for about 10 minutes, or until they're soft and warmed through. Mash them with the back of a wooden spoon until they have a jam-like texture. Transfer them to a bowl and refrigerate.

In a blender, purée the almond or coconut milk, peanut butter, optional honey or maple syrup, and optional collagen powder for 15 seconds, or until everything is well combined. Pour the liquid mixture into a large bowl. Sprinkle the chia seeds on top, then whisk them in well. Refrigerate the mixture for 2 hours. If you can, stir the pudding a couple of times while it's chilling. It will thicken as it sits. If it gets too thick, stir in a splash or two of additional almond or coconut milk.

To assemble the breakfast cups, divide half the chia pudding evenly between 4 small serving cups. Spoon in a layer of the chilled strawberries. Add a final layer of the chia pudding. If you'd like, top each with some chopped peanuts for crunch and/or fresh strawberries. Refrigerate the cups until you're ready to eat them.

Change It Up

– Swap almond butter for the peanut butter and make them AB and J cups!

– Use frozen blueberries instead of strawberries.

Sweet Potato Breakfast Bowls

GRAIN-FREE, DAIRY-FREE, EGG-FREE, NIGHTSHADE-FREE

As a kid, cereal was my favorite breakfast food. (I mean, who doesn't love the chocolate-y milk left over after a bowl of cocoa-flavored puffed cereal?!) Nowadays, I lean on protein and veggies as my breakfast mainstays, but from time to time, I still get a hankering for something a bit sweet. Enter my Sweet Potato Breakfast Bowls. With lots of fiber and slow-digesting carbs, these won't put you into a sugar coma. Plus, you can roast the sweet potatoes the night before to save time. Add in some collagen powder or serve with a side of eggs for a protein boost.

PREP TIME: 15 MINUTES
COOKING TIME: 45 MINUTES
SERVES 2 TO 4

2 pounds sweet potatoes, scrubbed
8 ounces bacon, baked
2 tablespoons coconut milk
1 teaspoon vanilla extract
Pinch of sea salt
2 tablespoons collagen powder, optional
1 pint fresh blueberries
1 ripe banana, sliced
¼ cup chopped almonds

Preheat the oven to 400°F.

Line a rimmed baking sheet with parchment paper. Place the sweet potatoes on the sheet and roast them for about 45 minutes, or until they're quite soft and a knife easily pierces through the flesh. Remove them from the oven, slice them open, and allow them to cool for a few minutes.

About 30 minutes into the roasting of the sweet potatoes, start baking the bacon (see page 256). Once the bacon is cool, roughly chop it, then set it aside.

To make the sweet potato purée, I find it easiest to cut the ends off the sweet potatoes, then peel the skin off. Place the roasted flesh into a food processor, then add the coconut milk, vanilla, salt, and, if desired, collagen powder. Purée for about 30 seconds, or until the mixture is smooth. If it's too thick, add a splash more of the coconut milk and process again. If you don't have a food processor, combine everything in a large bowl and stir it very well with a wooden spoon.

Divide the sweet potato purée between serving bowls. Top it with the chopped bacon, blueberries, sliced banana, and chopped almonds, and serve.

The bowls can be assembled ahead of time, but it's best to leave the fruit off until they're ready to eat. They can be eaten cold or gently reheated.

Change It Up

– Add a side of eggs for more protein.

– Make savory bowls with the same sweet potato purée but topped with sautéed spinach, sautéed mushrooms, bacon, and a fried egg.

Roasted Tomato and Garlic Soup

GRAIN-FREE, NUT-FREE, DAIRY-FREE, EGG-FREE

Soup is my food "love language," and nothing brings me back to childhood like a lunch of tomato soup and grilled cheese. Nowadays, I try to avoid canned soups because of their high sodium content and funky preservatives. Luckily, this homemade soup is simple to make. Roast the tomatoes ahead of time if you can. The coconut milk adds creaminess, and the fish sauce, a dash of savory umami. Top it with some crispy bacon and a little fresh basil. For a vegetarian version, use veggie broth and omit the fish sauce. And for a treat, pair this soup with a grilled cheese made from gluten-free bread and full-fat cheddar. Yum.

PREP TIME: 15 MINUTES
COOKING TIME: 40 MINUTES
SERVES 6

2 pounds ripe Roma tomatoes, quartered
1 sweet onion, roughly chopped
3 cloves garlic
4 to 6 sprigs fresh thyme
1 tablespoon olive oil
Generous pinch each of sea salt and ground black pepper
1 cup low-sodium chicken broth
2 tablespoons coconut milk
½ teaspoon fish sauce, optional

Preheat the oven to 400°F.

Line a rimmed baking sheet with parchment paper, and spread the tomatoes, onion, garlic, and thyme on the sheet. Drizzle them with the olive oil and sprinkle with the salt and pepper, then toss everything with your hands until it's well coated. Roast the veggies for 20 to 30 minutes, or until they begin to caramelize and brown around the edges. Remove the sheet from the oven.

Remove any leftover woody sprigs of thyme from the veggies, then add all the vegetables and garlic to a powerful blender or food processor. Pour in the chicken broth, then purée until the mixture is completely smooth, about 1 minute. (Be careful when blending hot liquids!)

Pour the blended mixture into a large pot set over medium heat. Stir in the coconut milk and optional fish sauce. Adjust the salt and pepper to taste. Let the soup simmer for 5 to 10 minutes, then serve it hot.

Change It Up

– Top the soup with shredded rotisserie chicken for a complete meal.

Hearty Tuscan Kale Soup

GRAIN-FREE, NUT-FREE, DAIRY-FREE, EGG-FREE

There's nothing like a hearty soup to warm the soul. And here's my secret: soup is one of my favorite ways to start the day. Yep, soup for breakfast. This one's filling, nourishing, and packed with veggies, and the chicken broth gives you a gut-soothing gelatin boost. Feel free to swap out the pork sausage for chicken. It'll be just as good. I like Yukon gold potatoes in this because they don't turn to mush like Idaho russets do. The key to this quick soup is to dice all the veggies the same size so everything cooks evenly.

PREP TIME: 15 MINUTES
COOKING TIME: 45 MINUTES
SERVES 4 TO 6

1 pound Italian pork sausage, removed from the casings
3 medium carrots, diced
2 large Yukon gold potatoes, peeled and diced
1 medium yellow onion, diced
2 cloves garlic, smashed with the side of a knife
½ teaspoon dried rosemary
6 cups low-sodium chicken broth
1 bunch green kale, tough stems removed, chopped
Sea salt and ground black pepper to taste

In a large pot or Dutch oven set over medium-high heat, brown the sausage, breaking the meat up with a wooden spoon, for about 5 to 7 minutes. Toss in the carrots, potatoes, onion, garlic, and rosemary. Give it all a good stir. Then pour in the chicken broth.

Cover the pot and raise the heat to high. Bring the soup to a boil, then reduce the heat and remove the lid. Simmer the soup for 15 to 20 minutes, or until the veggies are tender. Stir in the chopped kale, add salt and pepper to taste, and simmer for another 5 minutes, then serve.

Change It Up

– Trade the pork sausage for cooked shredded chicken.

– Add a can of white beans.

Fast Weeknight Pho

DAIRY-FREE, EGG-FREE

Pho is one of my favorite soups, a Vietnamese dish with richly spiced aromatic broth, rice noodles, fresh toppings, and any one of a variety of proteins. While I can't claim that this version of pho—pronounced "fuh"—is authentic, it's my homage to this humble but comforting dish, and one you can make quickly at home. I like pairing it with my Shrimp Yum Balls (page 283), but you could also top it with thinly sliced cooked steak or chicken. Feel free to use what you like as well as carb it up or down. You can always prep the broth on the weekend and reheat it later on for a super-fast dinner. Make it grain-free by using zucchini noodles instead of rice noodles.

PREP TIME: 30 MINUTES
COOKING TIME: 30 MINUTES
SERVES 2 TO 4

1 small yellow onion, halved
8 cups low-sodium beef broth
3 star anise
2 whole cloves
1 cinnamon stick
1 tablespoon coconut aminos
1 tablespoon fish sauce
2 cups rice noodles or zucchini
    noodles

Toppings

Mung bean sprouts
Lime, quartered
Fresh herbs (mint, cilantro,
    Thai basil, etc.)
Sliced jalapeño pepper
Chopped peanuts or cashews
Sriracha or chili oil

Preheat the broiler of your oven.

Line a rimmed baking sheet with foil, and place the onion halves on the sheet. Broil them for about 5 minutes per side, or until they've developed a little char, then remove them from the broiler, and transfer them to a large pot.

Add to the pot the broth, star anise, cloves, cinnamon, coconut aminos, and fish sauce. Bring the broth to a boil, then reduce the heat and simmer the pho for 20 to 30 minutes so the broth is infused with all the flavors. Turn off the heat, and use a slotted spoon to remove and discard the onion and spices.

Partially cook the rice noodles according to the package directions (they will finish cooking within the broth). If you prefer to "carb it down" with zucchini noodles, use them raw.

In each serving bowl, place the noodles of your choice, then ladle the broth over them, which will further cook your noodles.

Serve all the toppings on the table so each person can customize their soup as desired.

Change It Up

– Add any toppings or protein you'd like.

– In a pinch you can use chicken broth, but beef is more flavorful.

Fresh Spring Roll Salad with Ginger-Lime Dressing

DAIRY-FREE, NUT-FREE, EGG-FREE

This dish was inspired by my love for fresh spring rolls, and it's the perfect take-along lunch. Packed with protein and veggies, it's totally satisfying and full of flavor. Plus, you can carb this dish up or down by changing your choice of noodles. Choose rice noodles for a gluten-free version, or carb it down and keep it grain-free by using spiralized cucumber or zucchini noodles. Pack it into jars for ready-made portable meals.

PREP TIME: 20 MINUTES
COOKING TIME: 20 MINUTES
SERVES 4

1 8-ounce package rice noodles
1 pound chicken breasts or
    tenderloins
Generous pinch each of sea salt
    and ground black pepper
1 small napa or green cabbage,
    thinly sliced
¼ small red cabbage, thinly
    sliced
1 large carrot, thinly sliced
½ red bell pepper, stemmed,
    seeded, and thinly sliced
Optional garnishes: handful of
    fresh cilantro, handful of
    chopped cashews or peanuts,
    lime wedges

For the dressing
Juice of 2 limes
4 teaspoons coconut aminos
2 teaspoons rice wine vinegar
1 teaspoon freshly grated ginger
1 teaspoon sesame oil
¼ teaspoon fish sauce
1 clove garlic, finely chopped

Prepare the rice noodles according to the package directions, then set them aside to cool.

Place the chicken breasts in a large, high-sided skillet. Add the salt and pepper plus enough water to cover the chicken. Put a lid on the skillet, and bring the water to a boil, then reduce the heat to a simmer. Poach the chicken for about 15 minutes, or until it's completely cooked through, then transfer it to a plate to cool. When it's cool enough to handle, dice or shred it into small pieces.

In a medium bowl, combine all the ingredients for the dressing and whisk until it's well combined. Set it aside.

If you're serving the salad in bowls, place cooked rice noodles at the bottom of each bowl, followed by salad veggies, then chicken. Spoon the dressing over the top and top each bowl with the optional garnishes. If you're packing the salad into jars, spoon the dressing into the bottom, followed by the chicken, the noodles, the veggies, and any garnishes.

Change It Up

– Carb this dish down by swapping out the rice noodles for spiralized cucumber or zucchini noodles.

– Make the dressing creamy by whisking in a tablespoon of sunflower seed butter or peanut butter.

Steak Cobb Salad
with Southwestern Ranch Dressing

GRAIN-FREE, NUT-FREE, DAIRY-FREE

PREP TIME: 25 MINUTES
MARINATING TIME: 1 TO 8 HRS
COOKING TIME: 10 MINUTES
SERVES 4

Entrée salads for the win. The Cobb salad is an American classic, and this one has a twist. It's with marinated steak, crisp veggies, and a zingy southwestern ranch dressing. Make this salad ahead of time and portion it out for lunches, serve it up family style, or plate it individually—totally flexible.

For the steak

2 teaspoons ancho chili powder
½ teaspoon garlic powder
½ teaspoon ground cumin
½ teaspoon sea salt
¼ teaspoon dried oregano
¼ teaspoon dried thyme
¼ teaspoon ground black pepper
1 pound sirloin steak
Juice of 2 limes
Olive oil or ghee for cooking

For the salad

4 slices bacon
1 head green leaf lettuce, chopped
½ cucumber, peeled and chopped
½ pint cherry tomatoes, halved
½ small jicama, peeled and diced
2 ripe avocados, pitted and diced
2 hard-boiled eggs, peeled and
    quartered
2 ounces shredded full-fat
    cheddar cheese, optional
Cilantro and lime wedges, as
    garnishes

For the dressing

¼ cup avocado oil mayonnaise
Juice of 2 limes
1 tablespoon coconut milk
1 teaspoon ancho chili powder
½ teaspoon onion powder
½ teaspoon dried parsley
¼ teaspoon garlic powder
¼ teaspoon ground chipotle pepper
Sea salt to taste

In a small bowl, combine the ancho chili powder, garlic powder, cumin, salt, oregano, thyme, and black pepper. Place the steak in a large glass bowl or baking dish. Add the lime juice, then sprinkle the spice mixture on the steak. Massage the spices into the meat, and refrigerate the steak for at least an hour and up to 8 hours. (Great to do before leaving for work in the morning.)

While the steak is marinating, whisk together all the dressing ingredients in a medium bowl. Refrigerate the dressing until you're ready to use it.

Next, bake the bacon (see page 256), then chop it.

To assemble the salad, lay the lettuce on a large serving platter or serving plates. In rows, arrange the cucumber, tomatoes, jicama, bacon, avocados, eggs, and optional cheese.

Remove the steak from the marinade, letting any excess liquid drip off, and discard the marinade. Add about 1 tablespoon olive oil or ghee to a large cast-iron skillet set over medium-high heat. (I like ghee here because it has a higher smoke point than most oils.) When the pan is hot, sear the meat about 4 minutes on each side.

Remove the steak from the pan and place it on a cutting board to rest for at least 5 minutes. Then slice it and add the slices to the salad.

Drizzle the salad with the dressing, and garnish it with the chopped cilantro and/or lime wedges if you're feeling it.

Change It Up

– Top with avocado crema (from Loaded Taco Beef Nachos with Avocado Crema, page 276).

Spinach, Pear, and Pecan Salad with Balsamic Vinaigrette

GRAIN-FREE, DAIRY-FREE, EGG-FREE, NIGHTSHADE-FREE, VEGETARIAN

This dish reminds me of those fancy market salads that make me think, *I could make that at home*, so that's what I did. If you normally buy a grab-and-go salad for lunch, start making this one instead. It comes together so fast, and you know the ingredients are fresh. The key to bringing it all together is the homemade balsamic vinaigrette. Unlike those little packets of dressing you get alongside a market salad, this is made with good-for-you extra-virgin olive oil.

PREP TIME: 20 MINUTES
COOKING TIME: 5 MINUTES
SERVES 4

⅓ cup pecan halves
6 ounces baby spinach leaves
1 large pear, sliced
2 ounces soft goat cheese, crumbled, optional

For the vinaigrette
1 clove garlic
1 teaspoon dijon mustard
¼ cup balsamic vinegar
Pinch each of sea salt and ground black pepper
⅓ cup olive or avocado oil

First, make the vinaigrette. In a blender, purée the garlic, dijon mustard, balsamic vinegar, and salt and pepper for about 15 seconds, or until the garlic has broken down. While the blender is running, drizzle in the olive or avocado oil. If you don't have a blender, finely chop the garlic and whisk together all the ingredients except the oil in a large bowl. Then slowly drizzle in the oil while whisking. Easy peasy. Set the dressing aside.

In a small dry skillet set over medium-low heat, toast the pecans. Keep stirring them for about 3 to 5 minutes, or until the nuts are just lightly toasted. Be careful because these can burn in a flash! Then remove them from heat and transfer them to a bowl to cool.

In a large serving bowl, combine the spinach and sliced pear. If you're serving the salad right away, drizzle it with about half the dressing and toss well to coat everything. Taste the salad and add more dressing if you want. Top with the chopped pecans and optional goat cheese. If you'll be serving the salad later, top the spinach and pears with the toasted pecans and optional goat cheese, then dress it when you're ready to eat.

Any extra dressing can be stored in the fridge for up to a week.

Change It Up

– If you like your dressing less tangy, increase the olive or avocado oil to ½ cup.

– Top it with grilled chicken for a complete meal.

– Swap strawberries or blueberries for the pears.

– Substitute mixed salad greens for the spinach.

Chopped Broccoli Salad

GRAIN-FREE, DAIRY-FREE, EGG-FREE, NIGHTSHADE-FREE OPTION

This salad is one of those dishes that gets better when you let it sit overnight (though it's tasty right away too). Instead of traditional mayo-based dressings, which can weigh a salad down, I swapped in apple cider vinegar and olive or avocado oil. Carrots and blueberries add an antioxidant punch and a pop of color, the bacon adds a savory-salty note, the citrus zest adds some freshness, and the almonds bring a nice crunch. Serve it alongside your favorite protein for a complete meal.

PREP TIME: 20 MINUTES
COOKING TIME: 15 MINUTES
SERVES 6

8 ounces bacon
2 pounds broccoli crowns, finely chopped
2 cups fresh blueberries
2 medium carrots, grated
¼ cup chopped almonds
Zest and juice of 1 orange
¼ cup olive or avocado oil
2 tablespoons apple cider vinegar
Generous pinch of red pepper flakes, optional
Sea salt and ground black pepper to taste

Bake the bacon (see page 256). Once it's cool, roughly chop it, and set it aside.

While the bacon is baking, assemble the rest of the salad. In a large bowl, combine the broccoli, blueberries, carrots, almonds, orange zest, orange juice, olive or avocado oil, vinegar, and optional red pepper flakes. Toss everything well to combine. Top with the chopped bacon. Adjust the seasoning with salt and pepper.

Change It Up

– Swap out the chopped almonds for another nut.

– Use lemon juice and zest instead of orange.

– Leave out the red pepper flakes for a nightshade-free salad.

Roasted Carrots with Orange Dill Butter

GRAIN-FREE, NUT-FREE, EGG-FREE, NIGHTSHADE-FREE, VEGETARIAN

One of my fondest memories is pulling fresh carrots out of my grandfather's garden, running them under the backyard faucet, and munching on them on the spot. The humble carrot is loaded with beta-carotene, a powerful plant pigment that's converted by the body into vitamin A. I love carrots in all preparations, but my favorite is probably roasted because their natural sweetness really shines. Look for carrots on the thinner side—they'll roast faster. In this recipe, perfectly simple roasted carrots are topped with a tasty orange dill compound butter. Just four main ingredients!

PREP TIME: 10 MINUTES
COOKING TIME: 30 MINUTES
SERVES 4

2 bunches carrots (about 2
   pounds), washed, tops
   removed
1 tablespoon olive oil or melted
   ghee
Sea salt and ground black
   pepper to taste
2 tablespoons unsalted grass-
   fed butter, softened
¼ cup loosely packed fresh dill,
   chopped
Zest of 1 orange

Preheat the oven to 400°F.

Line a rimmed baking sheet with parchment paper. Spread the carrots on the sheet, drizzle them with the olive oil or melted ghee, and sprinkle them with a generous pinch of salt. Roast them for 25 to 35 minutes, stirring a couple of times, until the carrots are lightly browned and tender when pierced with a knife.

While the carrots are roasting, prepare the compound butter. In a medium bowl, combine the softened butter, dill, and orange zest. When the carrots are roasted, transfer them to a serving plate, and while they're still hot, dot them with the compound butter. Salt and pepper to taste.

Change It Up

– Use ghee instead of butter.

– Swap out the dill for parsley.

Cabbage, Bacon, and Noodles (Haluski)

GRAIN-FREE, NUT-FREE, EGG-FREE, DAIRY-FREE, NIGHTSHADE-FREE

My grandma Ruth always had a pot of something bubbling on the stove any time we went to visit her. Usually it was some kind of chicken soup or one of the Eastern European dishes she learned growing up. Grandma's father came through Ellis Island from Ukraine with his siblings and parents, and her mother was Polish. Needless to say, I grew up eating her pierogi, golumbki, kapusta, and simple variations of this cabbage, bacon, and noodle dish, known to many as haluski. To this day, these dishes are my comfort food and remind me of my grandma. To keep this recipe gluten-free, I use rotini noodles made from chickpea flour. Feel free to use any gluten-free noodles you like, or just leave them out. It'll still be delicious.

> PREP TIME: 10 MINUTES
> COOKING TIME: 30 MINUTES
> SERVES 4

8 ounces uncooked gluten-free chickpea rotini pasta

8 ounces bacon, chopped into ½-inch strips

1 medium yellow onion, sliced

1 medium green cabbage, cored and sliced into ribbons

Sea salt and ground black pepper to taste

Cook the pasta according to the package directions.

While the pasta is cooking, put the bacon in a large cold skillet. Set the skillet over medium heat and stir the bacon occasionally until the pieces begin to crisp, about 10 to 12 minutes.

To the same skillet, add the onion and cabbage. Stir everything so the veggies are coated in bacon fat and begin to soften. Continue to cook and stir until the cabbage and onion are soft and cooked through, about 15 minutes.

Turn off the heat. Add the pasta to the skillet, and stir everything until it's well combined. Taste and season it with salt and pepper if needed.

Change It Up

– Carb it down by omitting the gluten-free pasta.

Sautéed Kale with Balsamic Cherries

GRAIN-FREE, EGG-FREE, NIGHTSHADE-FREE, DAIRY-FREE, VEGETARIAN

The hat tip for this recipe goes to my dear friend Dallas, who introduced me to this delightful concoction. The savory garlic, tangy balsamic reduction, sweet-tart cherries, and crunchy pistachios make quite the combination! If kale isn't your thing, you could easily substitute chard or an equal amount of spinach. It's a more mouthwatering way to get your greens. It also makes a killer side dish to the Garlic Lamb Chops with Herb Gremolata (page 278).

PREP TIME: 10 MINUTES
COOKING TIME: 15 MINUTES
SERVES 4

1 tablespoon olive oil or ghee
2 cloves garlic, finely chopped
⅓ cup balsamic vinegar
½ cup dried tart cherries
2 bunches kale, tough stems removed, chopped
¼ cup shelled pistachios, chopped

In a large pot or Dutch oven set over medium heat, warm the olive oil or ghee. Then sauté the garlic for about a minute, until it smells scrumptious. Add the balsamic vinegar and cherries. Raise the heat, and bring the mixture to a boil, then lower the heat to medium-low, simmering 6 to 8 minutes or until the sauce is reduced by about half and the cherries are soft.

Add the kale to the pot and stir so it's well coated with the sauce. Cover and simmer until the kale softens, about 5 minutes. Serve the kale garnished with the pistachios.

Change It Up

– Swap the kale out for chard or spinach.

– Use walnuts instead of pistachios.

The Best Cauliflower Ever

GRAIN-FREE, EGG-FREE, DAIRY-FREE, VEGETARIAN

Cauliflower is one of the most underrated veggies out there, in my opinion. When roasted in the oven, it takes on a wonderfully nutty flavor. In this recipe, inspired by a dish at one of our favorite restaurants, it's roasted and tossed in a zingy sauce made from lemon, tahini (sesame seed butter), and harissa, a red pepper sauce. Then it's hit with some fresh herbs, chopped pistachios for crunch, and dried currants for a hint of sweetness. The result is damn delicious. Hint: I make a double batch because it disappears so fast.

PREP TIME: 10 MINUTES
COOKING TIME: 20 MINUTES
SERVES 4

1 medium or large head cauliflower, about 1½ to 2 pounds
1 tablespoon olive oil or melted ghee
Sea salt and ground black pepper to taste
Juice of 1 lemon
2 tablespoons mild harissa
1 tablespoon tahini
1 clove garlic, finely chopped
1 tablespoon chopped fresh mint
1 tablespoon chopped fresh parsley
¼ cup shelled pistachios, chopped
2 tablespoons dried currants or raisins

Preheat the oven to 400°F.

Cut the cauliflower florets off the core. I like to quarter the bigger florets so I get more flat surface area, maximizing the amount of yummy browned edges from roasting.

Line a rimmed baking sheet with parchment paper, and spread the cauliflower on the sheet. Drizzle the florets with the olive oil or ghee and sprinkle with a generous pinch of sea salt. Toss everything with your hands until it's well coated. Roast the cauliflower for about 20 minutes, stirring once or twice, or until the cauliflower is golden brown on the edges.

While the cauliflower is roasting, in a large bowl, mix the juice from a lemon with the harissa, tahini, and garlic. When the cauliflower is ready, toss it in the sauce. Add the chopped mint and parsley, then toss again. Adjust the salt and pepper to taste.

Serve it garnished with the pistachios and currants or raisins.

Change It Up

– Use chopped almonds instead of pistachios.

– No currants or raisins? No problem. Use dried cherries instead.

Roasted Root Veggies

GRAIN-FREE, NUT-FREE, EGG-FREE, DAIRY-FREE, NIGHTSHADE-FREE, VEGETARIAN

In the fall and winter, root veggies have my heart. Hidden inside their somewhat ordinary exteriors, they transform into magical veggie unicorns with a little heat, fat, and simple seasonings. This is my favorite mix of root veggies, but feel free to use what you have available in the market. The key to getting a tray of mixed veggies to cook evenly is to chop everything to roughly the same size. I like to keep the skins on all my root veggies—yay for extra fiber!—but feel free to peel them if you'd like. Sometimes I drizzle on a bit of my balsamic vinaigrette if I'm feeling fancy.

PREP TIME: 10 MINUTES
COOKING TIME: 40 MINUTES
SERVES 4 TO 6

3 carrots
3 parsnips
2 beets, red or golden
1 yellow onion
2 tablespoons olive oil or melted ghee
1 teaspoon dried parsley
1 teaspoon dried thyme
½ teaspoon ground black pepper
¼ teaspoon sea salt

Preheat the oven to 400°F.

Scrub the veggies, peeling them if you'd like. Roughly chop them, making sure the pieces are all about the same size.

Line a rimmed baking sheet with parchment paper, and spread the veggies on the sheet, then drizzle them with the olive oil or ghee. Sprinkle them with the parsley, thyme, pepper, and salt. Toss everything with your hands until it's well coated, and evenly distribute it all in one layer on the sheet. Roast the veggies for 40 to 45 minutes, stirring once or twice, or until they're tender and golden brown.

Change It Up

– Try other root veggies, like rutabaga or celery root.

– Sprinkle with fresh herbs—try rosemary or thyme—before serving.

Smoky Duck Fat Potato Wedges

GRAIN-FREE, NUT-FREE, EGG-FREE, DAIRY-FREE OR VEGETARIAN

There's nothing quite like roasted potatoes with their golden brown exterior and tender center . . . but when you roast them in duck fat, you take them to the next level. These potato wedges are tossed in smoked paprika and onion powder for the perfect smoky-savory flavor. If you can't find duck fat, try substituting ghee for a buttery finish. I really love Yukon gold potatoes for roasting because they have a smooth texture, thin skin, and beautiful yellow color.

PREP TIME: 10 MINUTES
COOKING TIME: 30 MINUTES
SERVES 4

1½ pounds Yukon gold potatoes
2 tablespoons duck fat or ghee, melted
1 teaspoon smoked paprika
1 teaspoon onion powder
½ teaspoon ground black pepper
¼ teaspoon sea salt

Preheat the oven to 400°F.

Scrub the potatoes. You can peel them if you'd like, but I usually don't. Cut the potatoes in half the long way, then into wedges.

Line a rimmed baking sheet with parchment paper, then spread the potatoes in one even layer on the sheet. Drizzle them with the melted duck fat or ghee, sprinkle them with the smoked paprika, onion powder, pepper, and salt, and toss them with your hands until everything is well coated. Roast them for 30 to 35 minutes, stirring once or twice, or until the potatoes are crispy and golden brown.

Change It Up

- Use red-skinned, white, or purple potatoes instead of Yukon gold.

- Sprinkle them with fresh herbs before serving—try parsley or chives.

Loaded Taco Beef Nachos with Avocado Crema

GRAIN-FREE, NUT-FREE, EGG-FREE, DAIRY-FREE

PREP TIME: 20 MINUTES
COOKING TIME: 15 MINUTES
SERVES 4

Olive oil or ghee for cooking
2 pounds grass-fed ground beef
2 tablespoons taco seasoning
1 teaspoon sea salt
5 to 6 ounces grain-free
    tortilla chips
3 Roma tomatoes, seeded and
    diced
½ red, yellow, or green bell
    pepper, stemmed, seeded,
    and diced
3 green onions, white and light
    green parts only, thinly sliced
¼ cup sliced black olives
4 ounces shredded full-fat
    cheddar cheese, optional
Large handful of fresh cilantro,
    chopped
1 lime, quartered

For the avocado crema

2 small ripe avocados,
    pitted and diced
2 tablespoons full-fat coconut
    milk
Juice of 1 lime
Small handful of fresh cilantro,
    chopped
¼ teaspoon sea salt
1 tablespoon pickled jalapeño
    rings, optional

Let's be honest: pretty much everyone loves nachos, but they're usually far from healthy, loaded with fake cheese and lacking in protein. This recipe is a better-for-you plate of nachos. I start with grain-free tortilla chips. (You can find them in many natural grocers or online.) Or you can roast thinly sliced sweet potatoes for your nacho base. Then top the base with grass-fed ground beef, fresh veggies, and a little shredded full-fat cheddar cheese.

Preheat the oven to 400°F.

In a large skillet set over medium-high heat, warm about a tablespoon of olive oil or ghee. Add the ground beef, and sprinkle it with the taco seasoning and salt. Break up the meat with a wooden spoon as it fries for about 6 to 8 minutes, until it's cooked through. Set the beef aside to cool as you make the crema.

In a food processor, purée all the ingredients for the avocado crema for about 30 seconds, or until the mixture is smooth. You may have to scrape down the sides with a rubber spatula and pulse a couple more times. No food processor? Use a fork to mash the avocado in a medium bowl, and stir in the rest of the ingredients until it's a smooth mixture.

Line a rimmed baking sheet with parchment paper. Layer your nachos on the sheet, starting with the tortilla chips, then adding the cooked beef. Use a slotted spoon to remove the beef from the skillet so you leave any excess fat behind. On top of the beef, add the tomatoes, bell pepper, green onions, and olives, and top with the optional cheese. Pop this into the oven for about 5 minutes, or until the cheese melts. Before serving, drizzle it with about half the avocado crema, and sprinkle it with chopped cilantro and a squeeze of lime. Save the other half of the avocado crema for the Steak Cobb Salad (page 267).

Change It Up

– Top the dish with black beans too.

Mini Meatloaf Sheet Tray Bake

GRAIN-FREE, NUT-FREE, EGG-FREE, DAIRY-FREE

Growing up, I was a lover of TV dinners and a hater of meatloaf. I don't eat TV dinners anymore, but this sheet tray bake reminds me of them a lot because you get a full entrée in one pan (minus the little fruit crumble dessert). Sheet tray bakes rock because there are no pots and pans to clean up afterward. The meatloaf has a bit of a kick from some ground chipotle peppers and smoked paprika, and the sweet potatoes and broccoli get perfectly roasted alongside. It turns out perfectly without bread crumbs or eggs as binders.

PREP TIME: 15 MINUTES
COOKING TIME: 50 MINUTES
SERVES 4

For the vegetables

3 small sweet potatoes, peeled and cut into ½-inch semicircles
Olive oil or melted ghee for cooking
Sea salt and ground black pepper to taste
1 pound broccoli florets

For the meatloaves

1 small red bell pepper, stemmed and seeded
½ small yellow onion
1½ pounds grass-fed ground beef
2 teaspoons dried parsley
1 teaspoon garlic powder
½ teaspoon ground chipotle pepper
½ teaspoon smoked paprika
1 teaspoon sea salt
½ teaspoon ground black pepper

Preheat the oven to 400°F.

Line a rimmed baking sheet with parchment paper, and spread the sweet potato semicircles on the sheet. Drizzle them with about a tablespoon of oil or melted ghee, and salt and pepper to taste. Toss the sweet potatoes with your hands until everything is well coated. Bake them for 10 minutes, then add the broccoli to the sheet, stirring it in with the sweet potatoes before returning the sheet to the oven for another 10 minutes.

While the vegetables are roasting, prepare the meatloaves. In a food processor, pulse the red bell pepper and onion until they're finely chopped but not a paste. You want the pieces to melt into the meatloaf. If you don't have a food processor, chop the red bell pepper and onion very finely with a knife.

In a large bowl, combine the red bell pepper and onion with the ground beef, parsley, garlic powder, chipotle pepper, smoked paprika, salt, and black pepper. Mix everything well with your hands, but don't overmix or the meat will become tough. Shape the mixture into four even mini loaves that are tapered at the edges.

After the broccoli has been roasting for its 10 minutes, move the veggies on the baking sheet to one side and add the meatloaves to the tray. Bake everything for 25 to 30 minutes, or until the mini meatloaves are cooked through.

Change It Up

– Use half ground beef and half pork for a lighter-tasting loaf.

Garlic Lamb Chops with Herb Gremolata

GRAIN-FREE, NUT-FREE, EGG-FREE, DAIRY-FREE, NIGHTSHADE-FREE

It wasn't until I took my first trip to New Zealand that I really started eating lamb. Now it makes a frequent appearance in our dinner lineup. For this recipe, the lamb is marinated in a generous amount of garlic and herbs, then pan roasted and topped with an herb gremolata. If you want, pop it into the fridge to marinate before you head to work in the morning. Traditionally, gremolata is a condiment made with lemon zest, garlic, parsley, and anchovies. I left the anchovy fillets out, but feel free to add them. These lamb chops make a killer accompaniment to The Best Cauliflower Ever (page 273).

PREP TIME: 15 MINUTES
MARINATING TIME: 2 TO 3 HOURS
COOKING TIME: 15 MINUTES
SERVES 4

2 pounds lamb chops (shoulder, or o-bone)
Sea salt and ground black pepper to taste
6 cloves garlic, smashed
4 sprigs fresh rosemary
¼ cup olive oil or avocado oil
Olive oil or ghee for cooking

For the gremolata
¼ cup chopped mint
¼ cup chopped parsley
1 clove garlic, finely chopped
Zest of 1 lemon
1 teaspoon olive oil
Pinch each of salt and ground black pepper

Lay the lamb chops on a plate or cutting board. Season both sides of them with salt and pepper. Place them in a baking dish with the garlic, rosemary, and olive or avocado oil. Massage the aromatics and oil into the meat, then let the chops marinate in the refrigerator for 2 to 3 hours, or overnight.

Preheat the oven to 400°F.

In a large oven-safe skillet set over medium-high heat, warm about a tablespoon of oil or ghee, but avoid letting it reach smoking temperature. Remove the meat from its marinade, shaking off any large pieces of garlic or herbs (they'll burn in the skillet and taste bitter). In the skillet, sear the lamb on one side for about 5 minutes, then flip them and place the skillet in the oven. Roast the chops for 7 to 10 minutes, depending on their thickness. Remove them from the oven and set them on a serving plate to rest for 5 to 10 minutes.

While the meat is resting, make the gremolata. In a small bowl, combine all the gremolata ingredients well, then spoon it evenly onto the lamb chops before serving.

Change It Up

– Use pork chops instead of lamb.

– Add fresh thyme to the marinade.

– Switch the lemon zest for orange in the gremolata.

Apple Braised Pork Shoulder

GRAIN-FREE, NUT-FREE, EGG-FREE, DAIRY-FREE, NIGHTSHADE-FREE

This scrumptious dish tastes like something that was complicated to make, but it's so simple. I've been making a version of this dish for years now, and it never disappoints. If you can let it cook low and slow in a Dutch oven, the meat becomes fall-apart tender in just a few short hours. You can also make it in an Instant Pot, which cuts the cooking time in half. And the apple juice naturally reduces into a perfect jus to spoon over the pork once it's done. For a veggie boost, nestle some cabbage wedges into the pot in the last hour of cooking.

PREP TIME: 5 MINUTES
COOKING TIME: 4 HOURS
SERVES 6

3 to 4 pounds pork shoulder or Boston butt, bone-in or boneless
Sea salt to taste
Olive oil or melted ghee for cooking
4 cups unsweetened apple juice
1 small green cabbage, cut into wedges, optional

Preheat the oven to 300°F.

Sprinkle the pork shoulder liberally with salt. In a Dutch oven or large oven-safe pot set over medium-high heat, warm about a tablespoon of olive oil or ghee. When the oil is shimmering, add the pork to the pot, searing one side for about 3 minutes, or until a nice golden crust develops. You'll know it's time to flip when the meat releases from the pan easily. Let the other side sear for about 3 to 5 minutes too, then turn off the heat and add the apple juice to the pot.

Put the lid on the pot and place it in the oven. After about 2 hours of roasting, you can add cabbage wedges to the pot if you like, then return it to the oven, covered, to roast for at least 1 more hour.

After 3 to 3½ hours, the meat will be super tender. Transfer it to a serving platter, then, using two forks, shred it. Place the cabbage wedges around it and spoon over some of the cooking liquid from the pot.

Change It Up

– Make this in a slow cooker. You'll need to reduce the amount of juice to 2 cups. Sear the meat as described, this time in a cast-iron skillet, then place the pork into the slow cooker and deglaze the skillet with about ¼ cup of the apple juice, scraping up any brown bits and adding that to the slow cooker too. Add the remaining 1¾ cups apple juice and cook the pork on low for 6 to 8 hours. In the final 2 hours, add the cabbage wedges if desired.

Chicken Tikka Masala

GRAIN-FREE, NUT-FREE, EGG-FREE

My husband is from Great Britain—Scotland to be precise—so he's eaten a ton of chicken tikka masala. When I first made this for him at home, I crossed my fingers it would make the cut. I anxiously asked, "So, what do you think?" He paused, quite dramatically, and exclaimed, "This is the best chicken tikka masala I've ever had!" Phew. If you're not familiar, chicken tikka masala is a very popular dish of marinated and then broiled or grilled chicken enrobed in a richly spiced tomato-based sauce. I swapped coconut milk for the traditional yogurt used in the marinade and the cream used in the sauce, and it's perfect.

PREP TIME: 20 MINUTES
MARINATING TIME: 60 MINUTES
COOKING TIME: 30 MINUTES
SERVES 4 TO 6

2 teaspoons garam masala
2 teaspoons ground coriander
2 teaspoons ground cumin
2 teaspoons ground turmeric
1 teaspoon sea salt
½ teaspoon ground black pepper
2 pounds chicken breast, cut into 1-inch chunks
1 14-ounce can full-fat coconut milk, divided (½ cup for the marinade and the rest for the sauce)
Juice of 1 lemon
2 cloves garlic, finely chopped
Cilantro for garnish

For the sauce

3 tablespoons ghee or grass-fed butter
1 medium yellow onion, finely chopped
1-inch piece fresh ginger, finely grated
3 cloves garlic, finely chopped
1 14-ounce can tomato sauce
Approximately 6 ounces full-fat coconut milk (the remainder from the marinade)
1 teaspoon fish sauce, optional
Sea salt to taste

In a small bowl, combine well the garam masala, coriander, cumin, turmeric, salt, and pepper. Set the spice mix aside.

Place the chicken in a baking dish or a large bowl, then add the coconut milk, lemon juice, and garlic, and sprinkle it with half the spice mix, combining everything well. Marinate the chicken in the refrigerator for about an hour, ideally.

In a large heavy-bottomed skillet set over medium heat, warm the ghee or butter until it's hot, then add the remaining half of the spice mix. Stir for about 30 seconds, until the spices are fragrant. Add the onion, ginger, and garlic, and sauté the mixture, stirring occasionally, until the onion is translucent, about 6 to 8 minutes. If the onion starts to brown, lower the heat. Add the tomato sauce, remaining coconut milk, and optional fish sauce, and salt to taste. Bring the sauce to a boil, then reduce the heat and simmer it for about 30 minutes, stirring often. The sauce will reduce by about a third. As the sauce is cooking, get the chicken cooking.

Preheat the broiler of your oven.

Line a rimmed baking sheet with foil, then place the marinated chicken on the sheet, shaking off excess marinade and discarding it. Broil the chicken until the edges are slightly charred, about 6 to 8 minutes. Don't let it burn! The chicken will still need a few minutes to finish cooking in the sauce.

Add the chicken to the simmering sauce and let it cook further for a few minutes. Adjust the seasonings if needed. Serve garnished with the cilantro.

Change It Up

– No broiler or grill? Bake the chicken in a 400°F oven for about 10 minutes, then add it to the sauce as described.

Honey Harissa Chicken Wings

GRAIN-FREE, NUT-FREE, EGG-FREE, DAIRY-FREE

Chicken wings make for a quick dinner on a weeknight because they basically cook themselves, leaving you free to catch up on chores. Plus, finger food is just more fun to eat, right?! Harissa is a North African sauce made from peppers, garlic, and smoky spices. Find it in the condiments aisle or online. These wings are quickly seared in a cast-iron skillet, basted with a spicy-sweet sauce, and finished in the oven. Serve it with steamed greens or a salad and a roasted sweet potato for a complete meal.

PREP TIME: 5 MINUTES
COOKING TIME: 30 MINUTES
SERVES 4

2 pounds chicken wings
Sea salt to taste
Olive oil or ghee for cooking
2 tablespoons mild harissa
2 tablespoons honey

Preheat the oven to 400°F.

Line a rimmed baking sheet with parchment paper, and place a metal baking rack on the baking sheet.

Pat the chicken wings dry with a paper towel, then sprinkle them on both sides with sea salt.

In a large cast-iron skillet set over medium-high heat, warm about a tablespoon of olive oil or ghee. When the oil is shimmering, add the chicken wings. Sear each side for about 5 minutes, or until a nice golden crust develops. You'll know it's time to flip when the meat releases from the pan easily. Remove the chicken wings and place them on the baking rack.

In a small bowl, combine the harissa and honey well, then brush the mixture on the chicken wings on all sides. If you have any of this sauce left over, you can baste the meat during baking.

Place the chicken wings on the baking sheet and bake for about 45 minutes, or until they are nice and crisp. Serve them hot.

Change It Up

– Serve the wings with extra honey harissa sauce for dipping—just be sure to mix a fresh batch that hasn't been in contact with raw chicken.

– Swap out the chicken wings for bone-in chicken thighs.

Greek Turkey Burgers

GRAIN-FREE, NUT-FREE, EGG-FREE, DAIRY-FREE, NIGHTSHADE-FREE

I always say that I should've been born in the Mediterranean because the food of Greece, Italy, and Spain really excites my palate. I love the briny olives, bright citrus, and pungent herbs, to name a few. The food is simple and rustic and speaks right to my heart. These Greek turkey burgers are my nod to the region, packed with fresh herbs, lemon, and red onion. The key to a perfect burger is to chop the added veggies finely. Serve these on lettuce wraps with your favorite toppings, on gluten-free buns, or on a salad for a complete meal.

PREP TIME: 15 MINUTES
COOKING TIME: 10 MINUTES
SERVES 6

2 pounds ground 93 percent lean turkey breast
1 cup packed fresh spinach leaves, finely chopped
¼ cup pitted black olives, finely chopped
Zest of 1 lemon
2 tablespoons finely chopped red onion
1 tablespoon finely chopped fresh mint or parsley
1 teaspoon garlic powder, or 3 fresh garlic cloves, finely chopped
1 teaspoon dried oregano
1 teaspoon sea salt
½ teaspoon ground black pepper
Olive oil or ghee for frying
Optional toppings: butter lettuce, sliced tomato, sliced red onion, sliced cucumber, more fresh mint or parsley, basil pesto (see Pesto Salmon Sheet Tray Bake, page 284), or feta cheese

In a large mixing bowl, use your hands to combine well the turkey meat with the spinach, olives, lemon zest, onion, mint or parsley, garlic, oregano, salt, and pepper. But don't over-mix or the meat will become tough. Divide the mixture into 6 equal portions and shape them into burgers.

Warm about a tablespoon of olive oil or ghee in a large skillet set over medium-high heat. Working in batches, add the burger patties and fry them on one side for about 5 minutes, then flip them, frying on the second side for another 4 to 5 minutes, or until they're golden brown.

If you like, serve each burger on a large piece of butter lettuce and top them with any of the optional ingredients.

Change It Up

– Serve these on top of a Greek-style salad.

– Swap out the turkey for ground chicken or lamb.

Shrimp Yum Balls

GRAIN-FREE, NUT-FREE, EGG-FREE, DAIRY-FREE, NIGHTSHADE-FREE

Sometimes naming recipes is hard. When testing recipes for this book, I'd give my husband the first bite. (He's notorious for saying exactly what's on his mind.) I gave him these meatballs and he asked, "What's in this?" I told him shrimp, and he replied, "Yum!" A man of many words. Thus the name Shrimp Yum Balls was born. Really, these are a mixture of ground pork and shrimp married with some of my favorite Asian flavors: ginger, green onion, and sesame oil. Totally reminiscent of the inside of a dumpling. I like to make a batch and toss them into my Fast Weeknight Pho (page 265) for a protein boost. My secret to fast, non-fussy meatballs is to scoop them with a disher, a scoop with a little release handle, and bake them.

PREP TIME: 15 MINUTES
COOKING TIME: 15 MINUTES
MAKES 18

8 ounces ground pork
8 ounces peeled and deveined shrimp (any size)
2 green onions, white and light green parts only, roughly chopped
1 small shallot, roughly chopped
½ teaspoon dark sesame oil
¼ teaspoon fish sauce
¼ teaspoon ground ginger
Generous pinch of ground black pepper
Sesame seeds and sliced green onion for garnish, optional

Preheat the oven to 375°F.

Line a rimmed baking sheet with parchment paper, and set it aside.

Put the ground pork in a large bowl and set it aside too.

In a food processor, combine the shrimp, green onions, shallot, sesame oil, fish sauce, ginger, and pepper. Pulse the mixture until the ingredients are broken down and no big chunks remain, but don't let it turn into a paste. Transfer the shrimp mixture to the bowl of ground pork, and use your hands to mix together everything well.

Using a 2 tablespoon disher or a large spoon, scoop the mixture into balls and set them on the prepared baking sheet. If you make them bigger or smaller, adjust the baking time accordingly. Pop the sheet into the oven and bake the balls for about 12 minutes, or until they're cooked through. Garnish them with sesame seeds and sliced green onion.

Change It Up

– Use all pork instead of the pork and shrimp combo.

– These freeze well.

Pesto Salmon Sheet Tray Bake

GRAIN-FREE, EGG-FREE, DAIRY-FREE

I'm all about the one-pan dinner. You get a complete hot meal, it basically cooks itself, and there are hardly any dishes to clean up. It's the perfect solution to a busy weeknight, because you can get in a home workout, tidy up the house, or watch some Netflix while it's baking. The salmon is topped with my dairy-free basil pesto for a punch of flavor. It's okay if the salmon skin is still on. The fish will detach effortlessly after it's cooked.

PREP TIME: 15 MINUTES
COOKING TIME: 45 MINUTES
SERVES 4

12 ounces fingerling potatoes, halved lengthwise
Olive oil or melted ghee for cooking
Sea salt and ground black pepper to taste
8 ounces green beans, ends trimmed
1½ pounds salmon, cut into 4 equal pieces

For the basil pesto

3 cups packed basil leaves (about 2 large bunches)
¼ cup pine nuts
2 cloves garlic
Juice of 1 lemon
6 tablespoons extra-virgin olive oil
Sea salt and ground black pepper to taste

Preheat the oven to 400°F.

Line a rimmed baking sheet with parchment paper, and spread the halved potatoes on the sheet. Drizzle them with about a tablespoon of olive oil or ghee, and sprinkle them with a generous pinch each of salt and pepper. With your hands, toss the potatoes so they're well coated. Bake them for 15 minutes.

Remove the sheet from the oven, add the green beans, stirring them around a bit to coat them in the oil, and return the sheet to the oven for another 15 minutes.

While the beans are cooking, make the pesto. In a food processor, combine the basil, pine nuts, garlic, and lemon juice, and pulse the mixture several times, until the big chunks are broken down. Then turn the food processor on and slowly add the olive oil. Taste and adjust the seasonings with salt and pepper. You'll use about ¼ cup of the pesto for this recipe. Store the rest in the refrigerator (it will last about three days).

Remove the sheet of vegetables from the oven. Make room on the tray for the salmon, adding it skin side down. Spoon about 1 tablespoon of the pesto onto each piece, then return the baking sheet to the oven for about 12 to 15 more minutes. Thinner pieces of salmon will need less time.

Change It Up

– Swap out the fingerling potatoes for sweet potato wedges.

– Not into salmon? Use any firm whitefish, and cut the cooking time down to about 10 to 12 minutes.

Bone Broth Latte

GRAIN-FREE, NUT-FREE, EGG-FREE, NIGHTSHADE-FREE, DAIRY-FREE OPTION

Bone broth is a great way to start your day off with a warm, nourishing boost of collagen. I love to blend mine with grass-fed butter and collagen powder for a creamy texture. If you're trying to decrease your coffee consumption, you can't have caffeine, or you're looking to switch up your morning routine, this warm and comforting drink just might do it. Be sure to drink it alongside a full meal.

PREP TIME: 5 MINUTES
COOKING TIME: 5 MINUTES
SERVES 2

2 cups low-sodium chicken bone
   broth; homemade is best
2 teaspoons grass-fed butter,
   ghee, or coconut milk
2 tablespoons collagen powder,
   optional
Pinch of sea salt

In a small saucepan set over high heat, warm the bone broth until it just starts to boil. Pour the heated broth into a blender, and add the butter, ghee, or coconut milk as well as the collagen and salt. Blend the mixture on high for 15 to 20 seconds, or until the broth is frothy and creamy. Serve immediately.

Change It Up

– Add 2 teaspoons matcha.

– Swap out the bone broth for 1 cup full-fat coconut milk or almond milk plus 1 cup water.

Creamy Golden "Milk"

GRAIN-FREE, NUT-FREE, EGG-FREE, DAIRY-FREE, NIGHTSHADE-FREE

Contrary to its name, this "milk" contains no dairy. What it does have is a bunch of nutritional power-houses together in a warm, creamy drink that's bound to satisfy. This recipe gets its rich golden color from ground turmeric, a spice popular in Indian cuisine that's known for its anti-inflammatory proper-ties. When you combine it with a healthy fat—found here in the coconut—and a little bit of black pepper, the anti-inflammatory compound curcumin is more easily absorbed by your body. This drink is infused with cinnamon and cardamom, lightly sweetened with honey, and frothed for the perfect latte foaminess. The collagen powder adds an optional protein boost.

PREP TIME: 5 MINUTES
COOKING TIME: 10 MINUTES
SERVES 2

2 cups full-fat coconut milk
2 cups water
1 tablespoon ground turmeric
¼ teaspoon ground ginger
1 cinnamon stick
4 cardamom pods, lightly crushed with the side of a knife
1 tablespoon honey
Generous pinch of ground black pepper
Pinch of sea salt
2 tablespoons collagen powder, optional

In a small saucepan set over high heat, warm the coconut milk, water, turmeric, ginger, cinnamon, cardamom, honey, pepper, and salt until the mixture just starts to boil, then reduce the heat and simmer it for about 10 minutes to let the spices really infuse the mixture.

Use a slotted spoon to remove the cinnamon stick and cardamom pods, and discard them. Pour the heated golden milk into a blender. Add the collagen if desired. Blend the milk on high for 15 to 20 seconds, or until it's frothy and creamy. Serve immediately.

Change It Up

– Swap out the coconut milk for almond or cashew milk.

– Add maple syrup instead of honey.

Stay Connected

Years ago, I read the book *ReWork* by Jason Fried and David Heinemeier Hansson. At the end was a contact page that said—and I paraphrase—"We hope you liked this book and that it inspires you. Drop us an email, and let us know how it's going." I absolutely adored the book, and so I thought, *Why not? I'll email them, but I doubt anyone will reply.* Much to my surprise and delight, not long after I pushed SEND, I received a personal response from Jason Fried himself. It was then and there that I decided to do my best to reply back to everyone who gets in touch. You inspire me to keep doing my best work.

I love hearing from you, so drop me a line. Shoot me an email, visit the website, or reach out on Instagram. Join the online community, and stay connected. Together we achieve more than any of us can alone.

Website: stephgaudreau.com
Email: stephg@stephgaudreau.com
Instagram: instagram.com/steph_gaudreau
Online community: facebook.com/groups/hardertokillclub

Selected References

PILLAR 1: EAT NOURISHING FOODS

ABC News Staff. "100 Million Dieters, $20 Billion: The Weight-Loss Industry by the Numbers." ABC News. May 8, 2012. https://abcnews.go.com/Health/100-million-dieters-20-billion-weight-loss-industry/story?id=16297197.

Baumeister, R. F., E. Bratslavsky, M. Muraven, and D. M. Tice. "Ego Depletion: Is the Active Self a Limited Resource?" *Journal of Personality and Social Psychology* 74, no. 5 (1998): 1252–65.

Baumeister, R. F., K. D. Vohs, and D. M. Tice. "The Strength Model of Self-Control." *Current Directions in Psychological Science* 16, no. 6 (2007): 351–55.

Calder, P. C. "N-3 Polyunsaturated Fatty Acids, Inflammation, and Inflammatory Diseases." *The American Journal of Clinical Nutrition* 83, suppl. 6 (2006): 1505S–1519S. doi: 10.1093/ajcn/83.6.1505S.

Council on Size and Weight Discrimination. "Statistics on Weight Discrimination: A Waste of Talent." Accessed July 18, 2011. http://www.cswd.org/index.html.

Duraffourd, C., F. DeVadder, D. Goncalves, F. Delaere, A. Penhoat, B. Brusset, F. Rajas, D. Chassard, A. Duchampt, A. Stefanutti, A. Gautier-Stein, and G. Mithieux. "Mu-Opioid Receptors and Dietary Protein Stimulate a Gut-Brain Neural Circuitry Limiting Food Intake." *Cell* 150, no. 2 (2012): 377–88.

Gailliot, M. T., R. F. Baumeister, C. N. DeWall, J. K. Maner, E. A. Plant, D. M. Tice, L. E. Brewer, and B. J. Schmeichel. "Self-Control Relies on Glucose as a Limited Energy Source: Willpower Is More than a Metaphor." *Journal of Personality and Social Psychology* 92, no. 2 (2007): 325–36.

Grodstein, F., R. Levine, L. Troy, T. Spencer, G. A. Colditz, and M. J. Stampfer. "Three-Year Follow-Up of Participants in a Commercial Weight Loss Program: Can You Keep It Off?" *Archives of Internal Medicine* 156, no. 12 (1996): 1302–6.

Gustafson-Larson, A. M., and R. D. Terry. "Weight-Related Behaviors and Concerns of Fourth-Grade Children." *Journal of American Dietetic Association* 92, no. 7 (1992): 818–22.

Inzlicht, M., and J. Gutsell, "Running on Empty: Neural Signals for Self-Control Failure." *Psychological Science* 18, no. 11 (2007): 933–37.

Job, V., C. S. Dweck, and G. M. Walton. "Ego Depletion—Is It All in Your Head? Implicit Theories About Willpower Affect Self-Regulation." *Psychological Science* 21, no. 11 (2010): 1686–93.

Martijn, C., P. Tenbült, H. Merckelbach, E. Dreezens, and N. De Vries. "Getting a Grip on Ourselves: Challenging Expectancies About Loss of Energy After Self-Control." *Social Cognition* 20, no. 6 (2002): 441–60.

Muraven, M., and R. F. Baumeister. "Self-Regulation and Depletion of Limited Resources: Does Self-Control Resemble a Muscle?" *Psychological Bulletin* 126, no. 2 (2000): 247–59.

National Eating Disorders Association. "Statistics: Eating Disorders and Their Precursors." Accessed February 2012. http://www.nationaleatingdisorders.org/uploads/statistics_tmp.pdf.

Neumark-Sztainer, D. *I'm, Like, SO Fat!* New York: Guilford Press, 2005.

Shisslak, C. M., M. Crago, and L. S. Estes. "The Spectrum of Eating Disturbances." *International Journal of Eating Disorders* 18, no. 3 (1995): 209–19.

Sundgot-Borgen, J., and M. K. Torstveit. "Prevalence of Eating Disorders in Elite Athletes Is Higher Than in the General Population." *Clinical Journal of Sports Medicine* 14, no. 1 (2004): 25–32.

University of North Carolina at Chapel Hill. "Three Out of Four American Women Have Disordered Eating, Survey Suggests." *ScienceDaily*, April 23, 2008. https://www.sciencedaily.com/releases/2008/04/080422202514.htm.

US Department of Health and Human Services, Centers for Disease Control and Prevention, and National Center for Health Statistics. *Health, United States, 2016: With Chartbook on Long-Term Trends in Health.* Washington, DC: US Government Publishing Office, 2017.

PILLAR 2: MOVE WITH INTENTION

Klok, M. D., S. Jakobsdottir, and M. L. Drent. "The Role of Leptin and Ghrelin in the Regulation of Food Intake and Body Weight in Humans: A Review." *Obesity Research* 8, no. 1 (2007): 21–34.

US Department of Agriculture, Agricultural Research Service. "Table 5. Energy Intakes: Percentages of Energy from Protein, Carbohydrate, Fat, and Alcohol, by Gender and Age." In *What We Eat in America, NHANES 2013–2014.* https://www.ars.usda.gov/ARSUserFiles/80400530/pdf/1314/Table_5_EIN_GEN_13.pdf.

US Department of Agriculture, Agricultural Research Service. "Table 25. Snacks: Percentages of Selected Nutrients Contributed by Food and Beverages Consumed at Snack Occasions, by Gender and Age." In *What We Eat in America, NHANES 2013–2014.* https://www.ars.usda.gov/ARSUserFiles/80400530/pdf/1314/Table_25_SNK_GEN_13.pdf.

US Department of Agriculture, Agricultural Research Service. "Table 37. Total Nutrient Intakes: Percent Reporting and Mean Amounts of Selected Vitamins and Minerals from Food and Beverages and Dietary Supplements, by Gender and Age." In *What We Eat in America, NHANES 2013–2014.* https://www.ars.usda.gov/ARSUserFiles/80400530/pdf/1314/Table_37_SUP_GEN_13.pdf.

PILLAR 3: RECHARGE YOUR ENERGY

Ahima, R. S., and H.-K. Park. "Connecting Myokines and Metabolism." *Endocrinology and Metabolism* (Seoul) 30, no. 3 (2015): 235–45.

Centers for Disease Control and Prevention. "Short Sleep Duration Among US Adults." https://www.cdc.gov/sleep/data_statistics.html.

Christensen, M. A., L. Bettencourt, L. Kaye, S. T. Moturu, K. T. Nguyen, J. E. Olgin, M. J. Pletcher, and G. M. Marcus. "Direct Measurements of Smartphone Screen-Time: Relationships with Demographics and Sleep." *PLoS One* 11, no. 11 (2016): e0165331. doi: 10.1371/journal.pone.0165331.

Clark, B. C., and T. M. Manini. "What Is Dynapenia?" *Nutrition* 28, no. 5 (2012): 495–503.

Deloitte. "2017 Global Mobile Consumer Survey: US Edition: The Dawn of the Next Era in Mobile." https://www2.deloitte.com/content/dam/Deloitte/us/Documents/technology-media-telecommunications/us-tmt-2017-global-mobile-consumer-survey-executive-summary.pdf.

Júdice, P. B., M. T. Hamilton, L. B. Sardinha, and A. M. Silva. "Randomized Controlled Pilot of an Intervention to Reduce and Break-Up Overweight/Obese Adults' Overall Sitting-Time." *Trials* 16 (2015): 490.

Owen, N., A. Bauman, and W. Brown. "Too Much Sitting: A Novel and Important Predictor of Chronic Disease Risk?" *British Journal of Sports Medicine* 43, no. 2 (2009): 81–83.

Seguin, R. A., G. Eldridge, W. Lynch, and L. C. Paul. "Strength Training Improves Body Image and Physical Activity Behaviors Among Midlife and Older Rural Women." *Journal of Extension* 51, no. 4 (2013): 4FEA2.

Tabata, I., K. Nishimura, M. Kouzaki, Y. Hirai, F. Ogita, M. Miyachi, and K. Yamamoto. "Effects of Moderate-Intensity Endurance and High-Intensity Intermittent Training on Anaerobic Capacity and VO2max." *Medicine and Science in Sports and Exercise* 28, no. 10 (1996): 1327–30.

PILLAR 4: EMPOWER YOUR MIND

Bank of America Corporation. *Trends in Consumer Mobility Report 2015*. https://www.scribd.com/document/269996235/2015-BAC-Trends-in-Consumer-Mobility-Report-Chicago.

Deloitte. *Global Mobile Consumer Survey 2016: UK Edition*. May–June 2016. http://www.deloittestore.co.uk/Mobile-Consumer-Survey-2016-p/mcs2016nfs.htm.

Forsythe, P., J. Bienenstock, and W. A. Kunze. "Vagal Pathways for Microbiome-Brain-Gut Axis Communication." *Advanced Experiments in Medicine and Biology* 817 (2014): 115–33.

Gorlick, A. "Media Multitaskers Pay Mental Price, Stanford Study Shows." Stanford News Service, August 24, 2009. https://news.stanford.edu/2009/08/24/multitask-research-study-082409/.

Green, A., M. Cohen-Zion, A. Haim, and Y. Dagan. "Evening Light Exposure to Computer Screens Disrupts Human Sleep, Biological Rhythms, and Attention Abilities." *Chronobiology International* 34, no. 7 (2017): 855–65.

Motomura, N., A. Sakurai, and Y. Yotsuya. "Reduction of Mental Stress with Lavender Odorant." *Perceptual and Motor Skills* 93, no. 3 (2001): 713–18.

WEEK 2: SETTLE IN

Simpson, S. J., and D. Raubenheimer. "Obesity: The Protein Leverage Hypothesis." *Obesity in Review* 6, no. 2 (2005): 133–42.

WEEK 3: HIT YOUR STRIDE

Geraerts, E., D. M. Bernstein, H. Merckelbach, C. Linders, L. Raymaekers, and E. F. Loftus. "Lasting False Beliefs and Their Behavioral Consequences." *Psychological Science* 19, no. 8 (2008): 749–53.

Gratitude

There's an old cliché that says writing a book takes a village, but it really is true. It's humbling to reflect on how many freaking incredible souls have been instrumental in the making of this work. You have inspired me, counseled me, nudged me, and given me the realest of real talk that it took to step out of my comfort zone and do something new.

On a personal level, I have the best support system on the planet. My husband, Z . . . you endured me reading you countless drafts, brainstormed so many titles, and had my back through many tough decisions. Your advice, eye for good writing, and tea-making skills are second to none. I love you. My family, you're a patient and supportive bunch. Even though I've been the obstinate black sheep intent on blazing a different path in life, you have never once said my dreams were crazy.

This book wouldn't have happened without the support of Sydney Rogers, Gideon Weil, and the HarperOne family . . . I feel seen, valued, and respected in your eyes. Thank you for helping bring the vision of this book to life and thus, positively affecting the lives of women all around the world. Dado Derviskadic and Steve Troha, my ever-patient and loving agents . . . what a journey! I'm forever grateful that you stuck with me for all these years and helped me mold this book into one that I am so proud of. (I promise that I know how to write a book proposal now!) And of course, to Kelly James, the best damn writer and integrator I could have hoped for. You kept me on

track, translated my rambles into something that made sense, and brought a can-do attitude to this project that I needed. Thanks, Warhammer. I couldn't have done this without you.

Next, I have so many friends to thank that listing you all would require more pages than I have left. You *all* have been instrumental in some way. Special gratitude goes out to: Jamie Scott, Anastasia Boulais, Dallas Hartwig, Melissa Joulwan, Kristen Roberts, Dr. Jolene Brighten, Aimée Suen, Julie Jones, Rachael Bryant, Ciarra Colacino, Amy Densmore, Dave Conrey, Theresa Larson, Beth Manos-Brickey, Kristen Boehmer, Meghan Hibner, Becky Greene, Brenda Swann, Lindsey Reeves, and Rick Santa Maria. To Richwell Correa and Taylor Gage, your artistry brought life to these pages. Your photography talents are unparalleled. And finally, Allegra Stein . . . what can I say? You've seen it all and been there for the whole ride. I'm lucky to have you in my life.

And finally, my readers and community, this is your book too. Thank you for the inspiration that's stoked the fires of my passion for health and wellness. Without you, none of this would exist. May it serve as the most delicious nourishment for your body, mind, and soul.

About the Author

Steph Gaudreau, NTC, BS, MA, gets up in the morning for one mission: to help women create bigger, bolder, *fiercer* lives—by building their health from the inside out. She's a bestselling author, Nutritional Therapy Consultant, women's health and fitness expert, podcaster, weightlifting coach, and blogger-photographer at StephGaudreau.com and the former StupidEasyPaleo.com. Her professional career began with a twelve-year run teaching high school biology and chemistry. In 2013, she left the classroom to help women learn how the right blend of nutrition, fitness, and mindset has the power to change their lives. Steph's other books are the award-winning *Performance Paleo Cookbook* and *The Paleo Athlete*.

Steph holds numerous fitness certifications, including USA Weightlifting Level 1 and many CrossFit certs. She lives in San Diego with the loves of her life, her husband, Z, and her cat, Ellie. When she's not lifting heavy stuff, you can find her tending to her garden, practicing Brazilian jiu-jitsu, and reading about how to be a better human.